MANAGING THE VIOLENT PATIENT
A Clinician's Guide

MANAGING THE VIOLENT PATIENT

A Clinician's Guide

Edited by

PATRICIA E. BLUMENREICH, M.D.

SUSAN LEWIS, R.N., C.S., Ph.D.

Routledge
Taylor & Francis Group
LONDON AND NEW YORK

First published 1993 by Brunner/Mazel, Inc.

2 Park Square, Milton Park, Abingdon, Oxon OX14 4RN
711 Third Avenue, New York, NY 10017, USA

Routledge is an imprint of the Taylor & Francis Group, an informa business

First issued in hardback 2016

Library of Congress Cataloging-in-Publication Data
Managing the violent patient : a clinician's guide / edited by Patricia E. Blumenreich, Susan Lewis.
p. cm.
Includes bibliographical references and index.
ISBN 0-87630-707-1
1. Violence in psychiatric hospitals. 2. Psychiatric hospital patients—Restraint. I. Blumenreich, Patricia E. II. Lewis, Susan (Susan Jane)
[DNLM: 1. Dangerous Behavior. 2. Nurse-Patient Relations. 3. Patients. 4. Psychiatric Nursing. WY 160 M266 1993]
RC439.4.M35 1993
616.85'8206—dc20
DNLM/DLC
for Library of Congress 93-12563
CIP

ISBN 978-0-87630-707-6 (pbk)
ISBN 978-1-138-16593-9 (hbk)

Dedicated to:

My husband, Martin
my daughters, Hannah and Arnina
my parents, Dr. Mendel Dulman and Elena Dulman—P.E.B.

The memory of my father, James O. Lewis
the "McKee Girls," Elizabeth, Mae, and Edna
my very special friend, Shangool—S.L.

Contents

Foreword

Violence is a growing concern in American life, with fear of dangerous behavior increasingly becoming a preoccupation in our society. Public interest in violence is developing into a major, even political issue, with instances of terrorism, spousal or child abuse, and date rape as pressing examples of recent concerns. Media attention is progressively more focused on dramatic acts of assault and homicide. Violence is seen in gang, cult, and mob activities; it occurs with organized groups, by individual random acts, and from the domestic environment. Etiologies for the increased frequency of such activities may include poverty, disenfranchisement, dissolution of the traditional family, and changes in social custom or mores. The easy availability of guns, graphic depictions of violence on television or movies, abuse of power, and diminished respect for authority figures all are said to enhance this trend. The attention of the nation clearly is directed toward this problem.

Violence has invaded the health care profession, too. Medical personnel have been victimized by threats, attacks, and other precarious experiences, similar to our culture at large. Gunfire in the emergency room or even at doctors' offices is no longer a very rare event. Concerns about this problem have made health care staff much more attentive to the risk involved and have driven many facilities to planning ways of preventing and managing the presence of dangerousness (e.g., providing greater protection with increased security surveillance).

Mental health professionals are also working at assuring the safety of their patients, staff, and themselves. Selected psychiatric patients may even have certain predispositions toward dangerousness. The arrival of this book, *Management of the Violent Patient*, in a time of so much concern for this topic, makes it indeed a welcome reference. The book provides a brief, concise source of information about preserving hospital and clinic safety through prevention and treatment.

Management of the Violent Patient is a multiauthored book, edited by Patricia E. Blumenreich, M.D., and Susan Lewis, R.N., C.S., Ph.D. It offers a comprehensive approach to a difficult clinical problem. The first four chapters provide a rich background into the epidemiology, etiology, and assessment of violent people from the medical point of view. Statistics on the risk for injury in health care facilities are illustrated. Characteristics of the victims, perpetrators, settings involved, and related aspects are presented for review. The etiology of dangerous behavior, from substance abuse implications to genetic predispositions and psychology, is nicely covered for the reader. Evaluation issues for the clinician are defined in a descriptive, practical manner.

The next four chapters addressing treatment cover interventions, pharmacotherapy, physical management of overtly dangerous individuals, and the application of seclusion and/or restraints. The verbal techniques have the potential of defusing threats, even before physical assault occurs. Recommendations for the use of drugs applies to prescribing both prophylactically for long-term treatment and acutely for immediate calmative action once menacing and/or combative instances emerge. A series of defensive and proactive maneuvers are detailed for teaching staff how to intervene in hazardous circumstances. Clinical and legal aspects of seclusion and restraint policies are delineated for the practitioner and administrator.

The final three chapters offer a change of pace to theoretical treatises about hostage situations, institutional reactions to violent acts prevention and management, and the legal implications involved. There is a discussion on hostage-taking, a subject of great prominence in recent times. The book recommends a course of action for facilities to help ensure that the institution and the people associated with it are safer. The delicate, yet critically important nuances in the law for the better protection of patient and staff rights are also described, rounding out the closing chapter.

For the active clinician and/or hospital administrator, this book affords a realistic, easy-to-read approach to the management of violent individuals. It thoroughly examines the pertinent aspects of each principal subject area. Readers will find this volume worthy of study and a help to their patients, co-workers, and themselves.

STEVEN B. LIPPMANN, M.D.
Louisville, KY
March, 1993

Acknowledgments

The editors wish to especially acknowledge the invaluable assistance and patience of Carol Ralph in the preparation of this manuscript. Special thanks also are due to Jim Kastner, Lynn Thomason, Rebecca Bowen, and Kathy Train from the Library Service, Veterans Affairs Medical Center, Louisville, Kentucky.

Contributors

Anthony G. Belak, J.D., Attorney at Law, District Counsel, U.S. Department of Veterans Affairs, Louisville, Kentucky

Patricia E. Blumenreich, M.D., Assistant Professor, Department of Psychiatry and Behavioral Sciences, University of Louisville School of Medicine; Staff Psychiatrist, Louisville Veterans Affairs Medical Center, Louisville, Kentucky

David Busse, J.D., Attorney at Law, Assistant District Counsel, U.S. Department of Veterans Affairs, Louisville, Kentucky

Theodore B. Feldmann, M.D., Associate Professor, Department of Psychiatry and Behavioral Sciences, University of Louisville School of Medicine, Louisville, Kentucky

Phillip W. Johnson, Ph.D., Clinical Assistant Professor, Department of Psychiatry and Behavioral Sciences, University of Louisville School of Medicine, Louisville, Kentucky

Susan Lewis, R.N., C.S., Ph.D., Psychiatric Nurse Clinical Specialist, Department of Veterans Affairs Medical Center, Louisville, Kentucky; Assistant Clinical Professor, Department of Psychiatry and Behavioral Sciences, University of Louisville School of Medicine, Louisville, Kentucky.

James M. Morrison, M.S.S.W., Supervisor, Social Work Service, Veterans Affairs Medical Center, Louisville, Kentucky

Danielle M. Turns, M.D., Professor, Department of Psychiatry and Behavioral Sciences, University of Louisville School of Medicine; *Former* Chief of Psychiatry, Louisville Veterans Affairs Medical Center, Louisville, Kentucky

"Now seest thou son," the kindly master said, "The souls of those whom wrath did overquell. . . ."

Dante, The Divine Comedy
Inferno Canto VII

1

Introduction

PATRICIA E. BLUMENREICH, M.D.
SUSAN LEWIS,
R.N., C.S., PH.D.

The incidence of violence in our society is on the rise. From 1989 to 1990 the overall rate of violent crime showed an increase of 11% (Index of Crime, 1990). This is an issue of importance for psychiatric professionals. Rates of assaultiveness and acting-out behavior are higher among psychiatric patients than previously thought. Some 33% to 40% of psychiatric admissions are preceded by violence (Parks, 1990). Assaultiveness in emergency psychiatric patients has been reported to be as high as 60% (Parks, 1990), although this figure may be somewhat lower in many settings.

Violence in psychiatric patients results from a complex interaction of multiple factors. Not only must the patient be considered in the context of the diagnosis or illness, but also in a broader perspective of physical, psychological, and sociocultural factors. The addition of immediate situational stress complicates matters further.

Patients generally are violent for identifiable reasons and give warning signals in advance of acting out. Clinicians can react to threats of personal harm in several ways. They can deny, ignore, or fail to recognize it, or they can freeze, panic, or respond therapeutically.

This book focuses on various aspects of dealing with disruptive patients. Guidelines for verbal, pharmacological, and physical intervention are discussed. Many of the physical management techniques presented in this volume are adapted from those originally developed by the Department of Veterans Affairs Medical Center and Physical Crisis Institute (PCI) in Cleveland, Ohio. When working with dangerous or potentially dangerous persons, *prevention* is the key. early intervention with interpersonal and/or chemical means can prevent a situation from erupting into physical violence.

Clinicians need to be able to recognize cues in the patient's history, physical condition, mental status, differential diagnosis, and behavior that indicate a potential for violence. And they must be aware of their own feelings of fear and anger that signal caution. Once this potential is identified, staff members need to know how to prevent violence and to minimize its damaging effects if violence should occur (Factor, 1991). No matter how skilled the practitioner, there is always a chance of injury to patients or staff members when physical contact takes place.

Knowledge of the principles of the prevention and management of disruptive behavior and thorough assessment tempered with common sense can avert a crisis. In emergency rooms, admitting areas, and other treatment units, the milieu should be structured to minimize risk. A warm, comfortable decor is more soothing. The area should be free of sharp and other objects that can be thrown or used as weapons. Escape routes should be accessible, as should ways of summoning additional staff. Crowding and noise should be kept to a minimum.

The staff members' demeanor should communicate respect, confidence, and a willingness to help. Both professionals and nonprofessionals need to be aware of ways in which they may provoke patients and ways in which they can defuse anger. The staff must be constantly "tuned in" to the level of tension in the clinical setting. Threats of harm to the patient's self or others should be taken seriously. A disturbed patient needs to be allowed expanded personal space.

Every treatment area should have policies and procedures specifying health and safety measures. There should be a sufficient number of well-trained staff members available to deal with possible crises. The presence of permanent staff members can facilitate the prevention of violence whereas the use of temporary staff can increase its likelihood (Haven & Piscitello, 1989). A prearranged signal to summon assistance should be designated. Ongoing training and review of techniques are essential. In addition, it is crucial that staff members function as a team when responding to violence.

After each incident, staff members should hold debriefing sessions. The object of these is not to place blame, but to evaluate what happened and improve methods.

It is difficult to predict violence over the long term; however, predictions of the potential for short-term violence can be fairly accurate. Diagnosis, a history of violence, the presence of drugs and alcohol, and current behavior can alert the clinician to the level of risk. The most effective way to deal with violent and/or assaultive behavior is to prevent it from ever happening.

REFERENCES

Factor, R. (1991). Managing the violent patient in the emergency department. *Emergency Care Quarterly,* 7(1), 82–93.

Haven, E., & Piscitello, V. (1989). The patient with violent behavior. In S. Lewis, R. Grainger, W. McDowell, R. Gregory & R. Messner (Eds.), *Manual of psychosocial nursing interventions* (pp. 187–204). Philadelphia: Saunders.

Index of Crime (1988). *Vital statistics of the United States* (DHHS Publication, Vol. 2, Part 18). Washington, D.C.: U.S. Government Printing Office.

Parks, J. (1990). Violence. In J.R. Hillard (Ed.), *Manual of clinical emergency psychiatry* (pp. 147–160). Washington, D.C.: American Psychiatric Press.

2

Epidemiology

DANIELLE M. TURNS, M.D.
PATRICIA E. BLUMENREICH, M.D.

Dangerousness has become a concern for our entire society, especially since crime has steadily increased in incidence over the past 30 years. The health professions have a stake in the issue as up to 50% of human services workers become victims of violence at some time during their careers. Deadly assaults on physicians are rare, but they raise community concerns, particularly if the assaulter is identified as a "mental patient."

Whether persons with a psychiatric disorder have more aggressive behavior than those without has long been a controversy. Studies linking violence and mental disorders have provided inconsistent results, partly because of methodological bias. What constitutes violence has been defined differently by different researchers—ranging from threats to actual crimes, including both violent and nonviolent acts. Some investigators have included individuals who were arrested for their crimes, whereas others have focused on only those who were convicted. Most often, perpetrators were identified as patients only if they had a history of contacts with the public mental health system where they had received a psychiatric diagnosis. A significant number of violent acts are never reported, and when they are, the offenders may not be arrested, or convicted, or even identified, decreasing the reliability of the data even further. For example, rapes are 50% unreported according to a police estimate; arrests are made in only half of the reported cases. Among those arrested, two thirds are prosecuted, with a 47% conviction rate. Therefore, 200 actual incidents may result in only 15 convictions (Rabkin, 1979). As for the identification of psychiatric patients, not all get into public health-care systems. Such characteristics as sex, age, race, socioeconomic status, and distance from services influence their entry into treatment (Jarvis, 1866). The same applies to severity of illness: individuals with psychosis, depression, and dementia are more likely to have received attention in public facilities, with aid from social and legal agencies. They are more likely to be arrested and convicted if involved in a crime, if only because of poor cooperation with their lawyers. These populations are not a true reflection of either dangerousness or mental illness.

The relationship between aggression and psychiatric disorders has been examined using data from a 1984 Epidemiologic Catchment Area Survey (Swanson, Holzer, Ganju, & Jono, 1990). Adult diagnoses were attained through responses to the Diagnostic Interview Schedule (DIS). To count as a positive case, the respondents had to meet the diagnostic criteria for a given disorder during the 12 months preceding the interview. Five specific questions on the DIS address violence:

1. Did you ever hit or throw things at your wife/husband/partner? (If so) were you ever the one who threw things first, regardless of who started the argument? Did you hit or throw things first on more than one occasion?
2. Have you ever spanked or hit a child (yours or anyone else's) hard enough to cause a bruise, injury, or need to see a doctor?
3. Since age 18, have you been in more than one fight that involved exchanging blows, other than those with your husband/wife/partner?

4. Have you ever used a weapon such as a stick, knife, or gun in a fight since you were 18?
5. Have you ever gotten into physical altercations while drinking?

Only violent episodes that occurred within 12 months were included in the study. The persons interviewed lived in the community and the diagnosis did not depend on a treatment, in order to avoid the entry of selection skew. Dangerousness was not assessed through arrests or conviction documents, but through personal disclosure. While self-reporting is not always accurate, such errors are thought to impart less systematic bias than do legal factors.

The results showed that the one-year incidence of violence in 10,059 persons interviewed was 3.7%, that is, 368 people responded positively to at least one item. Being male, young, and of low socioeconomic status was associated with aggressiveness. Men (5.29%) were more than twice as violent as women (2.2%), and people 18 to 29 years of age reported twice as much violence (7.3%) as the age group 30–44 (3.6%). Among people under 45, rates of violence were about three times higher for those in the lowest socioeconomic group than for those in the highest socioeconomic group.

Among the 368 violent responders, 55.5% met the criteria for a psychiatric disorder as compared with 19.6% of the non-violent persons. Substance abuse was identified 10 times more often among dangerous persons; affective disorders and schizophrenia were three times more common. The assessment of patients by diagnostic category reveals that the proportion of violence is relatively similar at about 11% across most diagnoses, except for phobia and substance abuse. Only 2% of the respondents with no psychiatric history admitted to violence; approximately 5% of phobic individuals reported dangerousness, and yet 25% of the substance abusers did. As to the type of assaults reported, hitting a child was the least common at 0.2% and fights with persons other than a spouse the highest (1.8%), and weapons were used in 1% of incidents. Striking a spouse was revealed by 1.4% and fighting while drinking also by 1.4%. Having had only one incident of combativeness was reported by 2.4%, and two or more incidents by 1.3%. No one admitted five or more occasions of dangerousness.

There is an almost linear relationship between the number of diagnosed conditions and the incidence of aggression: 2.1% for no diagnosis, 6.8% for one diagnosis, 17.5% for two diagnoses, and 22.4% for three or more. This may be indicative of any of the following: (1) polydiagnoses with significant psychopathologies that induce combativeness; (2) substance abuse, which heralds dangerousness; (3) endorsement of multiple symptoms associated with overreporting of violence; (4) use of psychiatric symptoms as an excuse for behavior; and (5) abuse of drugs in an attempt at self-medication. All five hypotheses probably contain some truth.

The question of the severity or frequency of violence and the severity or polymorphy of mental disorders has been addressed. In fact, 77% of the people with no psychiatric diagnosis who reported violence reported only one instance. About 50% of those with a psychiatric diagnosis answered positively on two or more items, hinting at a relationship between mental disorders and the frequency of aggression. Diagnoses with a high proportion of dangerousness, such as substance abuse, are associated with positive responses on multiple violence-related items.

In summary, there is clear evidence that people with mental disorders or substance-abuse problems report more assaultive behavior than do those without them. Anxiety and affective disorders, when they are the sole diagnosis, do not greatly increase the risk of aggression. Alcohol and substance abuse and the presence of more than one other diagnosis greatly elevate the risk. Aside from mental illness, male sex, young age, and lower socioeconomic status increase the chances of aggression substantially. People with schizophrenia do indulge in violence (12.7%), particularly if they are also drug abusers. When schizophrenia is the only diagnosis, the proportion falls to 8.4%. Since there are fewer schizophrenics than there are alcoholics in the population, citizens run a much larger risk of being attacked by an alcoholic than by a schizophrenic. These findings have important implications for community agencies, legal and judicial authorities, and mental health planners.

The information about the characteristics of dangerous patients in treatment has been gathered from a variety of settings, through different methods, and has yielded contradictory conclusions. Violent incidents in treatment settings tend to be underreported. In a Maryland state hospital, only 18% of assaults were formally reported (Lion, Snyder, & Merrill, 1981). Only 36% of "attacked" staff members filed a complaint (Thackey & Bobbitt, 1990). Aggression goes unreported, and milder behavior such as fear-inducing threats receives even less attention. Because of this underreporting, it is difficult to verify or impugn the commonly held belief that assaults are a small part of acting-out behavior.

PREVALENCE OF ASSAULTS

Data gathered from mental health professionals who had been victims of an attack by a patient and information about the frequency of assaults in institutions were documented in several investigations. The mental health professionals' reports on assaults vary from 5% to 50%. This variability is accounted for by methodological differences and response rates. The two studies with a 100% response rate (Madden, Lion, & Penna, 1976; Ruben,

Wolkon, & Yamamoto, 1980) gave a lifetime prevalence rate of 42% and a two-year incidence of 48%, which is particularly alarming since it concerns resident physicians-in-training. Later research gave an even higher rate of 63% (Gray, 1989). When only incidents resulting in bodily harm were included, a 5% positive response was obtained (Reid & Kang, 1986; Faulkner, Grimm, McFarland, & Bloom, 1990).

The treatment facilities' survey rates of assaults hover at around 10% at the time of or shortly after hospitalization and are even higher (21–38%) prior to admission. The rate of assault was found to be 2.5 per bed per year in psychiatric units, with the lowest rate in private facilities (1.2). State hospitals were in between with 3.3. In nonpsychiatric facilities, the rate is much lower (0.41), except for intensive care units (ICU), which had a substantial rate of 1.7 per bed per year, reflecting the acting out associated with delirium (Reid, Bollinger, & Edwards, 1985).

CHARACTERISTICS OF THE VICTIMS

There is a consensus among researchers (Whitman, Armao, & Dent, 1976; Bernstein, 1981; Carmel & Hunter, 1989) that the professional group most at risk is the nursing staff, followed by psychiatry residents and, finally, psychiatrists. This finding has not been verified for outpatient psychiatrists (Reid & Kang, 1986). Social workers and psychologists are victims less often. Family members are at highest risk, accounting for over 50% of the victims of patients who are violent prior to admission (Tardiff & Koenisberg, 1985).

The characteristics of the "attacked" mental health professional are not consistent or well defined: neither sex, age, race, nor the length of experience appears to be a discriminating factor. The risk for the psychiatrists has been reported by some to be higher early in their careers (Madden et al., 1976), while others have found no relationship (Dubin, Wilson, & Mercer, 1988). Among residents, no association with year of training was found because of confounding factors, such as the locus of rotation (Gray, 1989). No significant differences were noted for residents who had been assaulted only once; however, residents who had been hit more than once were characterized by a high irritability score, had expressed a willingness to fight if attacked, reported a high incidence of stressful events in the preceding weeks, and were in psychotherapy (Ruben et al., 1980).

All assaulted physicians felt that they had caused the attack by frustrating a patient's demands, by trying to impose medications or group attendance, or by being provocative in some way. Over half felt they should have anticipated the assault.

A positive relationship between the length of the therapy session and assault has been identified: 9% of the assaulted psychiatrists had never seen the patient, 10% were struck during the initial visit, 13% during the first month, and 36% after one year (Dubin et al., 1988). This trend may have contributed to the identification of insight-oriented psychotherapy as the most fertile area for aggression. Another hypothesis is that uncovering deep-seated conflicts and transference–countertransference issues may trigger violent acting out.

Nursing staff members tend to sustain more injuries while containing combative patients than by personal assault. Unit supervisors and senior psychiatric technicians are more likely to be injured during containment (Carmel & Hunter, 1989). Injuries among men about double those among women.

There are few large-scale reviews of patients assaulted by other patients. When this occurs, the victims are older than their assailants by an average of 16 years, lighter in weight, weaker or at most of equal strength, physically handicapped, and mentally disorganized. Usually they are of the same sex, males being overrepresented among both the strikers and the victims. Patients with neuroses, major affective disorders, and organic psychosis are more likely to be victims. Challenges to patient hierarchy on the ward and territoriality conflicts are believed to be precipitating factors (Depp, 1983).

CHARACTERISTICS OF THE ASSAILANTS

Research on the characteristics of assaultive patients does not yield consistent findings. Usually, age below 35 is associated more with violence, while 20% of geriatric patients assault someone prior to admission and another 20% indulge in fear-inducing behavior (Kalunian, Binder, & McNiel, 1990). Men are generally believed to be more violent than women. Males are more prone to assault prior to admission, but females are more dangerous after admission, during the early days of hospitalization (Binder & McNiel, 1990).

Schizophrenia is the disorder most frequently associated with combative behavior. Neurological and neuropsychological deficits in schizophrenic patients correlate with a high incidence of violence (Krakowski, Convit, Jaeger, Lin, & Volavka, 1989). Two different patterns of dangerousness among schizophrenics have been identified: Type I, occurring soon after admission, not associated with recidivism, quickly responsive to neuroleptics, and found in patients with a late onset of the disorder; and Type II, without a clear time course, associated with recidivism, less responsive to medications, and occurring in patients with an early onset of schizophrenia or some degree of neurological impairment (Volavka & Krakowski, 1989). Depressive affective disorders and mania do not demonstrate a consistent pattern. The substance abuse–violence relationship, so powerful in the community, does not appear so obvious once a person has been hospitalized. As for violent geriatric patients, senile dementia is the leading diagnosis (Kalunian et al., 1990; Balderston, Kelly, & Lion, 1990).

Demographic characteristics, such as race, socioeconomic status, and marital status, have not proved to be discriminating factors for violence in hospitalized patients. There is a general consensus that a previous history of combativeness is the best predictor of future dangerousness. Recidivists appear to be responsible for 53% of assaults. Suprisingly, female recidivists outnumber males, but they are less likely to induce serious harm. Young women with personality disorders are more likely to be repeat offenders, while schizophrenia increases the risk for males. Both men and women recidivists are younger than nonrecidivists (Convit, Isay, Ovis, & Volavka, 1990). Persistent offenders, however, represent a small proportion of the patients to whom one is exposed, so assessment will be biased if based only on that factor.

PLACE AND TIME

In general, outpatient settings such as mental health centers report a low rate of assault, but outpatient practitioners are not immune from risk. One study documented that 15 of 91 serious assaults and 17 of 59 less serious incidents took place in private office buildings, with eight and 15, respectively, in a hospital clinic; three of 91 and eight of 59 occurred at the psychiatrist's home (Dubin et al., 1988).

In hospitals, the emergency room is the most common site for violence, followed by ward corridors, dining or day rooms, and adolescent, child, and adult acute wards. Weapons are of particular concern in emergency rooms where 8.4% of patients were found to be carrying them (Anderson, Ghali, & Bansil, 1989).

As for time, the risk is highest at evaluation in the emergency room and during the first three days of hospitalization. Seasonal variations do not seem to affect assault rates; research has not verified the "full moon hypothesis" of mental illness–related violence on a monthly basis. The time of day shows no clear pattern. Incidents tend to cluster when patients have an opportunity to congregate and interact in crowded conditions. Therefore, findings vary greatly according to the type of institution and the scheduling of activities.

THE NATURE OF AN ATTACK

Assaults run the gamut from a simple shove to overt belligerence with the use of a deadly weapon: out of 68 assault cases, 85% involved blows to the head and body and 9% involved thrown objects, with the remainder divided among shooting, setting one on fire, tying the person up, and kissing (Madden et al., 1976). In another series of 91 attacks, there were 42 physical assaults, 17 incidents involving a gun, 15 involving a knife, and 17 involving thrown objects. The physical assaults induced 11 injuries and four cases of damage to property. None of the gun incidents resulted in physical or property damage, but two of the knife assaults caused property damage. Objects thrown did physical harm in three cases and property damage in five. It is interesting to note that gun situations lasted an average of 28 minutes (median 11); objects, 7.3 minutes (median 3); knives, 5.4 minutes (median 3); and physical assaults 5.4 minutes (median 1). Those incidents involving a gun perhaps lasted longer because of the degree of negotiation involved, while the other attacks had a lightning strike quality (Dubin et al., 1988).

WHY ATTACKS OCCUR

It is very important to determine what circumstances led to the violence. This is looked at in terms of the protagonists and the environment: the patient, the therapist, and the milieu.

As for the patients, there are clinical clues in addition to the diagnosis that are indications of impending danger. People showing high levels of thought disturbance, hostility, and agitation are more likely to be assaultive, regardless of the diagnosis (Lowenstein, Binder, & McNiel, 1990). Agressive individuals with a low level of anxiety are more likely to respond physically (Blomhoff, Seim, & Friis, 1990). An association between violence and emotional turmoil as manifested by agitation and anger has been described among schizophrenic, alcoholic, and organic patients. Males with other diagnoses were found to become assaultive in the absence of emotional distress; however, persons with affective disorders are unlikely to become assaultive even when angry or agitated (Craig, 1982). Neurological or neuropsychological deficits increase the likelihood of violence in schizophrenics (Krakowski et al., 1989). A history of familial violence should be heeded as a harbinger of the future. Threats involving unavailable parties are also dangerous since that anger may suddendly be displaced onto any present target (McNiel & Binder, 1989).

The therapeutic environment also plays a role in the development of potential attack, be it an institutional milieu or the classical patient–doctor dyad. Issues of staff response or expectations, conscious or unconscious conflicts, and transference and countertransference must all be examined.

Violence is often a reaction to overwhelming feelings of helplessness (Dubin, 1989). Hospital personnel, out of fear, may respond in an authoritarian or counteragressive manner, exacerbating the patient's feelings and precipitating acute combativeness. Staff members' anxiety or anger may lead to negative expectations of the patient's response to treatment and/or a rejecting stance. Overreaction to relatively minor acting out, punitive decisions, and excessive or lack of limit setting often result in violent situations. People with severe character pathology, noncompliance, and manipulative behavior enhance a divided staff potential for acting out its own anger and frustration. Conflicts among the staff members are "acted out" by patients (Stanton & Schwartz, 1954). Last, lower-level staff, through identification with the aggressor, may find some satisfaction in inciting a patient to attack an authority figure.

Countertransference issues such as frustration in reaction to a treatment-resistant patient may render the therapist unduly provocative. Unresolved conflicts about sex or aggression may result in punitive discharges, excessive limits on privileges, or unnecessary forced medications that are counterproductive to safety.

Denial is a powerful mechanism that can impede the gathering of clinically relevant information and prevent both the recognition of crucial danger "signals" and the undertaking of proper therapeutic action. Denial compounds unconscious omnipotent feelings such as, "No patient would attack me," and may even persist after the assault. In one study of outpatient psychiatrists, 59% continued to treat the perpetrator even if they had suffered injury, 21% never discussed the incident with the patient, and 33% made no change in the treatment plan or setting. Only 20% of them had any security system in place. In 66% of the cases, no change was made in the security system after experiencing a personal attack (Dubin et al., 1988).

IN CONCLUSION

Violence is a risk in one's personal life and professional career. Psychiatric patients are more likely than others to engage in fear-inducing or assaultive behavior. Even though the patient's own family members are the group most likely to be targeted, nurses and doctors are not immune from violence. Avenues of detection, prevention, and management of dangerous circumstances should be a priority of teaching programs, hospital administrators, and physicians.

REFERENCES

Anderson, A.A., Ghali, A.Y., & Bansil, E.K. (1989). Weapon carrying among patients in a psychiatric emergency room. *Hospital and Community Psychiatry, 40*(8), 845–847.

Armstrong, S. (1983). Assaults and impulsive behavior in the general hospital: Frequency and characteristics. In J.R. Lion & W.H. Reid (Eds.), *Assaults within psychiatric facilities* (pp. 119–130). Orlando, Fla.: Grune & Stratton.

Balderston, C., Kelly, G., & Lion, R.L. (1990). Databased interventions to reduce assaults by geriatric patients. *Hospital and Community Psychiatry 41*(4), 447–449.

Bernstein, H.A. (1981). Survey of threats and assaults directed toward psychotherapist. *American Journal of Psychotherapy, 35*, 542–549.

Binder, R.L., & McNiel, D.E. (1990). The relationship of gender to violent behavior in acutely disturbed psychiatric patients. *Journal of Clinical Psychiatry, 51*(3), 110–114.

Blomhoff, S., Seim, S., & Friis, S.V. (1990). Can prediction of violence among psychiatric patients be improved? *Hospital and Community Psychiatry, 41*(7), 771–775.

Bloom, J.D. (1989). The character of danger in psychiatric practice: Are the mentally ill dangerous? *Bulletin of the American Academy of Psychiatry and the Law, 17*(3), 241–255.

Carmel, H., & Hunter, M. (1989). Staff injuries from inpatient violence. *Hospital and Community Psychiatry, 40*(1), 41–46.

Convit, A., Isay, D., Ovis, D., & Volavka, J. (1990). Characteristics of repeatedly assaultive psychiatric patients. *Hospital and Community Psychiatry, 41*(10), 1112–1115.

Craig, T.J. (1982). An epidemiological study of problems associated with violence among psychiatric inpatients. *American Journal of Psychiatry, 139*, 1262–1266.

Depp, F.C. (1983). Assaults in a public mental health hospital. In J.R. Lion & W.H. Reid (Eds)., *Assaults within psychiatric facilities* (pp. 21–45). Orlando, Fla.: Grune & Stratton.

Dietz, P.E., & Rada, R.T. (1982). Battery incidents and batteries in a maximum security hospital. *Archives of General Psychiatry, 39*, 31–34.

Dubin, R.W. (1989). The role of fantasies, countertransference and psychological defenses in patient violence. *Hospital and Community Psychiatry, 40*(12), 1280–1283.

Dubin, R.W., Wilson, S.J., & Mercer, C. (1988). Assaults against psychiatrists in outpatient settings. *Journal of Clinical Psychiatry, 49*(9), 338–345.

Faulkner, L.R., Grimm, N.R., McFarland, B.H., & Bloom, J.D. (1990). Threats and assaults against psychiatrist. *Bulletin of the American Academy of Psychiatry and the Law, 18*(1), 37–46.

Gray, G.E. (1989). Assaults by patients against psychiatric residents at a public psychiatric hospital. *Academic Psychiatry, 13*, 81–86.

Haffke, E.A., & Reid, W.H. (1983). Violence against mental health personnel in Nebraska. In J.R. Lion & W.H. Reid, (Eds.), *Assaults within psychiatric facilities* (pp. 91–118). Orlando, Fla.: Grune & Stratton.

Hatti, S., Dubin, W.R., & Weiss, K.J. (1982). A study of circumstances surrounding patient assaults on psychiatrists. *Hospital and Community Psychiatry, 33*, 660–661.

Jarvis, E. (1866). Influence of distance from and nearness to an insane hospital on its use by the people. *American Journal of Insanity, 22*, 361.

Kalunian, D.A., Binder, R.L., & McNiel, D.E. (1990). Violence by geriatric patients who need psychiatric hospitalization. *Journal of Clinical Psychiatry, 51*(8), 340–343.

Katz, S.E., Cohen, R. & Stokman, C.L.J. (1985). Violence in psychiatric institutions. *New York State Journal of Medicine, 85*, 64–66.

Krakowski, M.I., Convit, A., Jaeger, J., Lin, S., & Volavka, J. (1989). Neurological impairment in violent schizophrenic inpatients. *American Journal of Psychiatry, 146*(7), 849–853.

Lagos, J., Perlmutter, K., & Saexinger, H. (1977). Fear of the mentally ill: Empirical support for the common man's response. *American Journal of Psychiatry, 134*, 1134–1137.

Lee, H.K., Villar, O., Juthani, N., & Bluestone, H., (1989). Characteristics and behavior of patients involved in psychiatric ward incidents. *Hospital and Community Psychiatry, 40*(12), 1295–1297.

Lion, J.R., Snyder, W., & Merrill, G.L. (1981). Underreporting of assaults on staff in a state hospital. *Hospital and Community Psychiatry, 32*, 497–498.

Lowenstein, M., Binder, R.L., & McNiel, D.E. (1990). The relationship between admission symptoms and hospital assaults. *Hospital and Community Psychiatry, 41*(3), 311–313.

Madden, D.J., Lion, J.R., & Penna, M.W. (1976). Assaults on psychiatrists by patients. *American Journal of Psychiatry, 133*, 422–425.

McNiel, D.E., & Binder, R.L. (1989). Relationship between preadmission threats and later violent behavior by acute psychiatric inpatients. *Hospital and Community Psychiatry, 40*(6), 605–608.

Noble, P., & Rodger, S. (1989). Violence by psychiatric inpatients. *British Journal of Psychiatry, 155*, 384–390.

Rabkin, J.G. (1979). The epidemiology of forcible rape. *American Journal of Orthopsychiatry, 49*(4), 634–647.

Reid, W.H., Bollinger, M.F., & Edwards, G. (1985). Assaults in hospitals. *Bulletin of American Academy of Psychiatry and the Law, 14*, 131–139.

Reid, W.H., & Kang, J.S. (1986). Serious assaults by outpatients or former patients. *American Journal of Psychotherapy, 40*, 594–600.

Ruben, I., Wolkon, G., & Yamamoto, J. (1980). Physical attacks on psychiatric residents by patients. *Journal of Nervous and Mental Disease, 168*, 243–245.

Sheridan, M., Henrion, R., Robinson, L., & Baxter, V. (1990). Precipitants of violence in a psychiatric inpatient setting. *Hospital and Community Psychiatry, 41*(7), 776–780.

Stanton, A.H., & Schwartz, M.S. (1954). *The mental hospital*. New York: Basic Books.

Swanson, J.W., Holzer, C.E., Ganju, V.K., & Jono, R.T. (1990). Violence and psychiatric disorder in the community: Evidence from the Epidemiologic Catchment Area Surveys. *Hospital and Community Psychiatry, 41*(7), 761–770.

Tardiff, K. (1984). Characteristics of assaultive patients in private hospitals. *American Journal of Psychiatry, 141*, 1232–1235.

Tardiff, K., & Koenisberg, H.W. (1985). Assaultive behavior among psychiatric outpatients. *American Journal of Psychiatry, 142*, 960–963.

Tardiff, K., & Sweillam, A. (1980). Assault, suicide and mental illness. *Archives of General Psychiatry, 139*, 164–169.

Tardiff, K., & Sweillam, A. (1982). Assaultive behavior among chronic inpatients. *American Journal of Psychiatry, 139*, 212–215.

Thackey, M., & Bobbitt, R. (1990). Patient aggression against clinical and non-clinical staff in a V.A. medical center. *Hospital and Community Psychiatry, 41*(2), 195–197.

Volavka, J., & Krakowski, M. (1989). Editorial: Schizophrenia and violence. *Psychological Medicine, 19*, 559–562.

Whitman, R.M., Armao, B.B., & Dent, O.B. (1976). Assault on the therapist. *American Journal of Psychiatry, 133*, 426–429.

3

Etiology

PATRICIA E. BLUMENREICH, M.D.

Violence is a phenomenon of multiple etiologies. It probably has many different interacting causes, involving both the individual's biopsychosocial background and environmental components. These factors interact in complex ways and are responsible for both repetitive acts and the isolated episode of aggression (Turpin, 1983). The nature of the setting has a powerful influence as a precipitant, facilitating or inhibiting an attack. Central nervous system (CNS) lesions, drugs, environmental stress, reinforcement, and modeling are causal elements in both human and nonhuman assaultiveness (Eichelman, Elliott, & Barchas, 1981).

PSYCHIATRIC DISORDERS

A psychiatric condition alone is not a good predictor of dangerousness, yet violence can result from the interaction between a patient and the environment. Under the proper circumstances, numerous conditions can be responsible for a patient's presenting with aggressive behavior. Predisposing factors plus current psychopathology and environmental elements codetermine whether an assault will occur. The psychiatric diagnosis most often associated with violence is acute schizophrenia, followed by personality disorders of the antisocial, borderline, explosive, and other types and organic brain syndromes. Other psychoses, mania, and depression can also cause one to exhibit dangerous behavior. The course of illness and symptomatology will affect the occurrence of violence. Characteristics of the episode will vary depending on the underlying situation. Young males with a family history of violence are the most likely to become assaultive. Many aggressive schizophrenic patients also suffer comorbidities with alcohol and/or drug abuse, seizure disorders, mental retardation, and so on, thus increasing the risk of violence.

Paranoia among schizophrenics fosters hazardous behaviors; their violent acts are usually well planned and consistent with their delusions. Such persons are more likely to commit a crime against family or friends and may cite vengeance as their motive (Krakowski, Volavka, & Brizer, 1986). The violence exhibited by disorganized, undifferentiated schizophrenic people is less focused and often less dangerous. Command hallucinations play a minor role in overt attacks. Delusional misidentification can also be associated with aggression. Various reports indicate that between 8% and 45% of schizophrenics are violent (Volavka & Krakowski, 1989). The estimates are so divergent because of the inconsistent definitions of violence, diagnostic criteria, patient selection, and settings.

Assaultive inpatients are likely to be young persons of both sexes diagnosed with schizophrenia, organic brain syndrome, mental retardation, or personality disorders. They are more likely than others to have a seizure disorder (Tardiff & Sweillam, 1982). Among the outpatients, diagnoses of childhood, adolescent, or personality disorders increase the risk of violent episodes (Tardiff & Koenigsberg, 1985). Patients with chronic conditions have the lowest incidence of physical aggression. Manic individuals are more likely to threaten than to assault, and they exhibit less criminality than do schizophrenics. In people with organic impairment, dyscontrol is unfocused and often less overt.

In personality disorders, hostility is a stable characteristic, present from an early age, not associated with emotional turmoil or any specific symptom cluster, and resistant to change. Consistent features in these individuals are histories of parental discord, divorce, separation, death, alcoholism, and abuse or neglect. Poor self-esteem and depressive traits are also present (Kay, Wolkenfeld, & Murrill, 1988).

In adolescents with conduct disorder, repetitive and severe offensive acts may indicate a special vulnerability of the nervous system, evidenced by episodic psychotic symptoms, limbic system dysfunction, cognitive impairment, or an abusive, violent family background (Lewis, Lovely, Yeager, & Della Femina, 1989).

Sleep-related violence is rare, but can be associated with a number of treatable sleep disorders. These include night terrors, sleepwalking, nocturnal seizures, rapid-eye-movement (REM) sleep behavior disorders, sleep drunkenness, and psychogenic, dissociative states occurring during sleep (Mahowald, Bundlie, Hurwitz, & Schenk, 1990).

DRUGS

Intoxication with many different substances can lead to violence. Common examples include alcohol, CNS depressants and/or stimulants, hallucinogens, and inhalants such as glue or paint. Alcohol withdrawal can also precipitate dangerous behavior. Alcohol, like other sedatives, may unmask inherent aggression (Bhattacharya & Datla, 1989). This effect is greatest among persons with a history of childhood aggression (Jaffe, Babor, & Fishbein, 1988). There is a clear causal relationship between alcohol consumption and assault. People who abuse alcohol commonly report more anger and hostility when drinking than when sober. Alcohol abusers, as a group, are more violence prone than are nonalcoholics, especially while drinking.

Alcohol and other sedatives facilitate emotional dyscontrol even more than they influence other behaviors (Bushman & Cooper, 1990). Individuals who consume alcohol are several times more likely than others to perpetrate physical attack or to be the victims (Norton & Morgan, 1989). Urban violence has been associated more with excessive binge drinking than with drug dependence, unemployment, or socioeconomic status (Shepherd, Robinson, & Levers, 1990). Patients who abuse alcohol and/or drugs, when not intoxicated or in withdrawal, are usually not dangerous in the hospital setting.

Research on the effects of cannabis is equivocal. It may not induce aggression under normal conditions, but it may do so under stress or frustration. The incidence of violence in chronic cannabis users is less than in phencyclidine abusers (Bhattacharya & Datla, 1989).

Narcotic addicts commit a vast amount of crime, much of it related to the need to purchase drugs (Nurco, Ball, Shaffer, & Hanlon, 1985). A great deal of this type of dangerousness is voluntary goal-directed activity as in a mugging. Violence is clearly associated with the use and abuse of cocaine. Many people who have met brutal deaths have been found to have cocaine in their bloodstreams and to have behaved in a dangerous manner prior to their death (Budd, 1989). Benzodiazepines also may have a disinhibiting effect similar to that of barbiturates or alcohol.

BIOLOGICAL DETERMINANTS

The present knowledge on the neurobiological basis of aggression has been gathered largely from animal research. It remains rudimentary and controversial and cannot be extrapolated to the human situation. Some theories have suggested that the ability to maintain empathy or sympathy is important in controlling combative behavior. Human belligerence can be inspired by frustration, anxiety, irritability, anger, depression, hatred, displacement, repression, prejudice, and animalization. It is generally accepted that environmental rather than genetic factors are important in the genesis of human assaultiveness (Bhattacharya & Datla, 1989). Aggression is controlled at multiple anatomical levels in the brain: hypothalamus, amygdala, septum, olfactory bulb, and orbital prefrontal cortex.

NEUROLOGICAL–ORGANIC FACTORS

Uncontrolled violent behavior is known to be one of the symptoms of structural brain damage. The chronic use of alcohol, vitamin deficiencies, tumors, infections, head trauma, and a lack of oxygen can upset the balance between the neocortex and limbic structures. As a consequence of anatomical brain disease, dangerous behaviors can occur. Nevertheless, many people with brain disease are not violent, and many dangerous individuals have no CNS lesion.

If the supply of oxygen fails at birth, the limbic system and especially the cells of the hippocampus are endangered. Other prominent causes of CNS damage include perinatal infections, prolonged reduction in blood sugar, severe cephalopelvic disproportion, Rh incompatibility, and/or physical damage to the baby's head during delivery.

Patients with injuries that mainly involve the temporal lobe are inappropriately combative as a result of limbic dysfunction. Other symptoms are difficulty in reading and speaking, disturbance in remote and recent memory, hallucinations, feelings of panic, and evidence of complex partial seizure disorders (Mark & Ervin, 1970). The underlying disorder in the limbic system, particularly the temporal lobe, is the one that is etiologically related to impulsivity and aggression. Temporal lobe convulsions are only one symptom of such malfunctioning. Complex partial seizures (CPS) have been related to violence, but not all patients with epilepsy are so inclined, or even demonstrate poor impulse control. Seizures do not generally induce dangerousness (Mark & Ervin, 1970).

Brain dysfunction affecting the limbic system is more apt to be related to emotional dyscontrol than disease in other areas of the brain, and many such patients exhibit structural or functional psychiatric disorders. Menacing individuals with emotional dyscontrol often share four historical characteristics: physical assault, especially toward a spouse or child; pathological intoxication; impulsive sexual behavior, including sexual attacks; and numerous traffic violations or serious automobile accidents. Violence, sex crimes, and dangerous driving often coexist (Mark & Ervin, 1970). Recognition and diagnosis are essential for appropriate therapy. Violence may be preventable in certain instances in people with treatable malfunctioning brain pathology.

The relationship between electroencephalographic abnormalities arising from the limbic system and dangerousness remains unclear. Aggression has been reported as one of the changes evidenced during the interictal period and has also been associated with dementia (Devinsky & Bear, 1984).

Among nursing-home residents, individuals with significant cognitive impairment may manifest aggression (e.g., hitting) and physical non-assaultive behaviors (e.g., pacing) (Cohen-Mansfield, Marx, & Rosenthal, 1990). Extreme aggression in some brain-damaged persons is regarded as an involuntary neural dysfunction that results from frontal lobe dysfunction (Gedye, 1989).

Other organic causes of violence may be related to toxic elements. The lead and cadmium contents in hair have been reported to be significantly higher in a group of violent incarcerated criminals when compared with nonviolent prisoners (Pihl & Ervin, 1990). Violent individuals are documented as having altered calcium–zinc, calcium–iron, copper–iron and iron–manganese ratios as compared with the population in general. There is also a relationship between lead and cadmium levels and hyperactivity, behavioral problems, and aggression in children.

NEUROTRANSMITTERS

No single chemical regulator has a unique signal for violence. Those that are important in controlling aggression also influence other important behaviors. Several neuroregulators, including dopamine (DA), norepinephrine (NE), acetylcholine (AC), and serotonin (5-HT), have specific functions in the initiation and execution of assault. The role of specific transmitters may depend on the type of aggression being studied. Dopamine and NE act similarly by facilitating and inhibiting responses. Activation of the cholinergic system induces both predatory and affective aggression, while the serotonergic system appears to be inhibitory for both. There seems to be an increase in plasma concentration of phenylethylamine metabolites in violent prisoners when compared with nonviolent controls. In military personnel, with both passive and aggressive-impulsive behavior, a direct correlation between dangerousness and cerebrospinal fluid (CSF) levels of 3-methoxyhydroxyphenilglycol and an inverse relationship between 5-hydroxyindoleacetic acid (5-HIAA) and aggressive scores have been documented (Eichelman et al., 1981).

With regard to serotonergic function, altered (5-HT) responsivity is probably associated with assaultiveness and dysphoria but not with impulsivity (Moss, Yao, & Panzak, 1990). However, relatively low 5-HIAA concentrations were found in the CSF of impulsive violent criminal offenders, as opposed to those whose acts were premeditated. Other CSF monoamines or metabolite concentrations were not significantly different between the groups. Impulsive aggressive offenders who had attempted suicide had the lowest 5-HIAA levels. A low concentration of

5-HIAA in the CSF may be a marker of impulsivity rather than of dangerousness (Linnoila, Virkkunen, Scheinin, Nuutila, Rimon, & Goodwin, 1983).

Attempts to correlate HIAA levels in CSF with measures of aggression in nonhuman primate species have alternately revealed an inverse, direct, or no correlation. A mixed serotonin 1A-B agonist and a more selective 1B agonist specifically decreased violence in several animal species (Meltzer, Linnoila, Miczek, Mos, & Olivier, 1989). Animal researchers who investigated gamma-aminobutyric acid (GABA)–mediated feline aggression concluded that gabaminergic mechanisms are selectively involved in the regulation of affective behavior at the level of the midbrain periaqueductal gray area (Shaikh & Siegel, 1990).

GENETICS

Genetic abnormalities had been thought to predispose to violent behavior, but the chromosomes themselves do not directly influence such actions. There is little compelling evidence to support theories of inherited factors in human aggression. People with a genetic abnormality are not uniformly violent or antisocial. A specific karyotype may be a predictor of brain malfunction, perhaps at a limbic system level, and disturbed behavior probably is related to altered brain function (Mark & Ervin, 1970). The XYY configuration, though, does seem to be related to antisocial behavior, especially violence; people with this finding appear to be more refractory to social rehabilitation than are criminals with the XY karyotype. The XXY profile is significantly represented in criminal and mental institutions; it occurs in 4% of male inmates as compared with 0.2% in the general population.

On the other hand, a study of 4591 men with XYY and XXY documented through clinical interviews, projective testing, and social records showed that they were not particularly violence prone. The XYY group had an increase in the concentration of testosterone, luteinizing hormone (LH), and follicle-stimulating hormone (FSH); the XXY subjects had an increase in FSH and LH but had low testosterone. When divided into delinquent with and without violent conviction and nondelinquent, a significant increase in testosterone levels was seen among the aggressive ones (Schiavi, Theilgaard, Owen, & White, 1984).

There is a high rate of criminal activity among individuals born to a criminal parent. While violent XY persons usually had siblings who had broken the law, XYY males came from law-abiding families. Among 47 XYY and 47 XXY men, one study documented an increase in the crime rate and a decrease in intelligence, but failed to find an increase in violence. Criminality may be associated with low intelligence (Eichelman, et al., 1981). How genetic influences interact with environmental factors during development to facilitate or inhibit criminal and aggressive tendencies is not fully understood (Eichelman, et al., 1981).

THE THEORIES

Psychological–Psychoanalytic

Aggression is considered an instinctive, inherent part of human nature, a fundamental state, need, or drive (Barchas, 1981). Aggression and hostility are considered responses to anxiety, a way to overcome obstacles and to manage everyday life tasks (Roberts, Mock, & Johnstone, 1981).

Ethological

Disruptive behavior is instinctual, spontaneous, and the result of philogenetic processes (Roberts et al., 1981). The predisposition to aggression is largely inborn, but there is a complex interaction of heredity and environment.

Frustration–Aggression

According to this theory, aggression follows frustration. The existence of frustration leads to violence whose goal is injury to another organism or its surrogate.

Social Learning

Aggressive behavior is learned or acquired from one's personal background. Family influences, subculture contacts, and symbolic modeling are the major sources. Learning is also accomplished by direct experience.

Cultural Factors

Some cultural attitudes may sanction or even encourage violence in given situations (Levy, Salagnik, Rabinowitz, & Neumann, 1989). For this reason, the word "aggression" does not become synonymous with "illness." Other cultures discourage violence and promote the manifestation of less aggressive behaviors.

Developmental Factors

Growing up in an emotionally distant or disorganized family with poor structure and boundaries predisposes to violence. The same applies to childhood abuse victims. Similar factors include records of fighting, truancy, cruelty to animals, fire setting, and/or bedwetting (Levy et al., 1989).

Physical Factors

There is a relationship between heat and aggression. Moderately uncomfortable temperatures increase belligerence, while more extreme discomfort decreases it. Other physical stressors, such as foul odors, appear to influence hostile acts in a similar fashion (Bell & Baron, 1981).

CONCLUSION

Violence in psychiatric patients may be the consequence of multiple, different interrelated factors. These include not only a particular illness and its predisposition to aggression, but also elements that range from cultural background to substance abuse and biological or developmental influences. Awareness of these facilitating components can be important in the treatment of a violent individual.

REFERENCES

Barchas, P. (1981). Vantage points for viewing aggression. In D.A. Hamburg & M.B. Trudeau (Eds.), *Biobehavioral aspects of aggression* (pp. 17–26). New York: Liss.

Bell, P.A., & Baron, R.A. (1981). Ambient temperature and human violence. In P.F. Brain & D. Benton (Eds.), *Multidisciplinary approaches to aggression research* (pp. 421–430). New York: Elsevier-North Holland Biomedical Press.

Bhattacharya, S.K., & Datla, K.P. (1989). Aggressive behavior–basic and clinical frontiers. *Indian Journal of Medical Research*, *90*, 387–406.

Budd, R.D. (1989). Cocaine abuse and violent death. *American Journal of Drug and Alcohol Abuse*, *15*(4), 375–382.

Bushman, B.J., & Cooper, H.M. (1990). Effects of alcohol on human aggression: An integrative research review. *Psychological Bulletin*, *107*(3), 341–354.

Cohen-Mansfield, J., Marx, M.S., & Rosenthal, A.L. (1990). Dementia and agitation in nursing home residents: How are they related? *Psychology and Aging*, *5*(1), 3–8.

Devinsky, O., & Bear, D. (1984). Varieties of aggressive behavior in temporal lobe epilepsy. *American Journal of Psychiatry*, *141*, 651–656.

Eichelman, B., Elliott, G., & Barchas, J. (1981). Biochemical, pharmacological, and genetic aspects of aggression. In D.A. Hamburg & M.B. Trudeau (Eds.), *Biobehavioral aspects of aggression* (pp. 51–84). New York: Liss.

Gedye, A. (1989). Episodic rage and aggression attributed to frontal lobe seizures. *Journal of Mental Deficiency Research*, *33*, 369–379.

Jaffe, J.H., Babor, T.F., & Fishbein, D.H. (1988). Alcoholics, aggression, and antisocial personality. *Journal of Studies on Alcohol*, *49*(3), 211–218.

Kay, S.R., Wolkenfeld, F., & Murrill, L.S. (1988). Profiles of aggression among psychiatric patients. 1. Nature and prevalence. *Journal of Nervous and Mental Disease*, *176*(9), 539–546.

Krakowski, M., Volavka, J., & Brizer, D. (1986). Psychopathology and violence. *Comprehensive Psychiatry*, *27*(2), 131–148.

Levy, A., Salagnik, I., Rabinowitz, S., & Neumann, M. (1989). The dangerous psychiatric patient. Part I: Epidemiology, etiology, prediction. *Medicine and Law*, *8*, 131–136.

Lewis, D.O., Lovely, R., Yeager, C., & Della Femina, D. (1989). Toward a theory of the genesis of violence: A follow-up study of delinquents. *Journal of the American Academy of Child and Adolescent Psychiatry*, *28*, 431–436.

Linnoila, M., Virkkunen, M., Scheinin, M., Nuutila, A., Rimon, R., & Goodwin, F.K. (1983). Low cerebrospinal fluid 5-hydroxyindoleacetic acid concentration differentiates impulsive from non-impulsive violent behavior. *Life Sciences*, *33*, 2609–2614.

Mahowald, M.W., Bundlie, S.R., Hurwitz, T.D., & Schenck, C. (1990). Sleep violence—forensic science implications: Polygraphic and video documentation. *Journal of Forensic Sciences*, *35*(2), 413–432.

Mark, V.H., & Ervin, F.R. (1970). *Violence and the brain*. New York: Harper & Row.

Meltzer, H.Y., Linnoila, M., Miczek, K.A., Mos, J., & Olivier, B. (1989). Serotonin, aggression and self-destructive behavior. Brain 5-HT and inhibition of aggressive behavior in animals: 5-HIAA and receptor subtype. *Psychopharmacology Bulletin*, *25*(3), 399–403.

Moss, H.B., Yao, J.K., & Panzak, G.L. (1990). Serotonergic responsivity and behavioral dimensions in antisocial personality disorder with substance abuse. *Biological Psychiatry, 28*, 325–338.

Norton, R.N., & Morgan, M.Y. (1989). The role of alcohol in mortality and morbidity from interpersonal violence. *Alcohol and Alcoholism, 24*(6), 565–576.

Nurco, D.N., Ball, J.C., Shaffer, J.W., & Hanlon, T.E. (1985). The criminality of narcotic addicts. *Journal of Nervous and Mental Disease, 173*(2), 94–102.

Palmstierna, T., & Wistedt, B. (1989). Risk factors for aggressive behavior are of limited value in predicting the violent behavior of acute involuntarily admitted patients. *Acta Psychiatrica Scandinava, 81*, 152–155.

Pihl, R.O., & Ervin, F. (1990). Lead and cadmium levels in violent criminals. *Psychological Reports, 66*, 839–844.

Roberts, T.K., Mock, L.A., & Johnstone, E.E. (1981). Psychological aspects of the etiology of violence. In J.R. Hays, T.K. Roberts, & K. Solway (Eds.), *Violence and the violent individual* (pp. 9–33). Manchester, N.H.: Luce.

Schiavi, R.C., Theilgaard, A., Owen, D., & White, D. (1984). Sex chromosomes anomalies, hormones, and aggressivity. *Archives of General Psychiatry, 41*, 93–99.

Shaikh, M.B., & Siegel, A. (1990). GABA-mediated regulation of feline aggression elicited from midbrain periaqueductal gray. *Brain Research, 507*, 51–56.

Shepherd, J.P., Robinson, L., & Levers, B.G.H. (1990). Roots of urban violence. *Injury, 21*, 139–141.

Tardiff, K., & Koenigsberg, H.W. (1985). Assaultive behavior among psychiatric outpatients. *Americal Journal of Psychiatry, 142*(8), 960–963.

Tardiff, K., & Sweillam, A. (1982). Assaultive behavior among chronic inpatients. *American Journal of Psychiatry, 139*(2), 212–215.

Turpin, P. (1983). The violent patient: A strategy for management and diagnosis. *Hospital and Community Psychiatry, 34*(1), 37–40.

Volavka, J., & Krakowski, M. (1989). Editorial: Schizophrenia and violence. *Psychological Medicine, 19*, 559–562.

4

Assessment

PATRICIA E. BLUMENREICH, M.D.

A violent person is someone who behaves or acts in such a way as to produce physical harm or destruction (Lion, 1987). This American Psychiatric Association task force report definition from 1974 emphasizes the physical aspects of aggression; however, verbal aggression in the form of insults, loudness, and threats usually precedes an actual attack. The clinician should be aware of the characteristics of the violent patient in order to make an adequate assessment and quickly plan an appropriate therapeutic intervention.

The individual's demeanor indicates the immediate potential for acting-out behavior; one must be attentive to this and the emotions that it evokes. "Gut" feelings have to be taken seriously, and denial—that is, "This could never happen to me" —must be recognized. Doctors often become overconfident when trying to manage a violent person, thus endangering themselves or others. A realistic appraisal of the circumstances is of paramount importance when trying to prevent a violent outburst.

ANAMNESTIC ISSUES

The expression of aggression, whether verbal or physical, correlates best with the patient's background and partially with the medical diagnoses. The best candidate is a young male with a prior history of violence, regardless of his psychiatric status or diagnosis. The severity of illness, the specific diagnosis, and personality traits are poor predictors of violence potential (Monahan, 1988). Recent stressors, such as the loss of a significant other or a job, in an individual who tends to act out and has poor coping skills or problem-solving abilities can precipitate an overt aggressive instance.

Persons with certain specific psychiatric disorders, such as psychoses, some personality disorders (i.e., antisocial or borderline), and organic brain disorders (i.e., delirium, dementia, organic personality disorders), tend to present more frequently with violent symptomatology, which should alert the physician. Substance misuse can induce aggression during both intoxication and withdrawal states.

Anamnestic issues of relevance include the possession of weapons and occasions when used, the serving of prison or jail terms, and the existence of police records of assault and/or murder. A history of physical, sexual, and verbal abuse is always investigated. Those with a history of that particular trauma may be abusers, but may not act out in a hospital setting.

The assessment of potential violence includes three components: the patient, the interviewer, and the environment.

The Patient

A history of aggression in young psychotic men who have been hospitalized in the past is an excellent predictor of future outbursts (Smith & Hucker, 1991). The patient's behavior in the immediate past and the clinical presentation at the time of evaluation are better predictors of imminent violence than are the diagnosis and the chronic characteristics (Beck, White, & Gage, 1991). It is imperative always to consistently evaluate the following.

1. At present
   - possession of weapons: on self or readily available (i.e., in the car or home).
   - plans to use them.
   - Prospective victim(s): Is the person "angry at the whole world," or is there a particular individual or group identified for attack?
   - psychoactive substances: Is there evidence of intoxication or withdrawal?
2. Recent
   - losses (job, relationships)
3. Past history:
   - head trauma or seizures
   - childhood record of physical, sexual, verbal abuse
   - childhood reports of fire setting, cruelty to animals, truancy
   - military experience
   - extent and severity of previous episodes of violence
   - jail, prison terms and police record
   - charges pending
4. Mental status examination
   - Certain signs and symptoms are indicative of imminent attack and the clinician must quickly recognize them in order to try to prevent injury.
5. Appearance:
   - Tense, angry facies, clenched fists, menacing stance
6. Speech:
   - Loudness, profanity, threats
7. Affect:
   - Labile, constricted in anger
8. Mood:
   - Angry, hostile, agitated
9. Psychotic features:

    - Delusions (paranoid, grandiose), menacing hallucinations
10. Cognitive functions:
    - Disorientation
    - Impaired judgement, insight.

The Interviewer

The clinician has to recognize such feelings as anger and fear in order to react appropriately when confronted with violent people. These individuals can arouse many different emotions that will vary depending on the doctor's background and personality, as well as on such current issues as degree of job satisfaction and stressors (i.e., illness, personal loss). A patient's perception of the interviewer as hostile, threatening, or arrogant may precipitate an attack. Body language and speech can be interpretated by a susceptible patient as an invitation to act out or to calm down. A tense, angry stance with menacing speech on the part of a frightened clinician may be more dangerous than a relaxed but controlled posture, with a soothing but firm voice and straightforward communication. Denial can have devastating consequences since any health-care professional can be a victim.

The Setting

Those settings that appear to be cold or chaotic in the eyes of a patient may be more conducive to violence (Haven & Piscitello, 1989). Unclear staff members' roles and unpredictable schedules also can trigger dangerous behavior (Katz & Kirkland, 1990).

The tolerance for emotional dyscontrol will differ in various institutional settings and among individuals on the staff. On occasion, patients may be perceived as more dangerous than they really are if they are disliked by the staff and become the recipient of projected anger (Lion, 1987).

Mixed-gender wards, poorly structured activities, and crowded areas have been identified as environmental characteristics conducive to attacks (Rice, Harris, Varney, & Quinsey, 1989). A decrease in the permanent nursing staff with a subsequent increase in temporary agency personnel is correlated with more violent incidents (James, Fineberg, Shah, & Priest, 1990).

When choosing the setting where a patient will be evaluated, the clinician needs to be aware of items that could be used for attack and for self-protection (see Chapter 5 on Verbal Intervention).

CONCLUSIONS

The results of research on the risk assessment of violence are inconsistent, ranging from studies that report an increase in predictive accuracy to those that indicate that a risk assessment is no better than chance (Monahan, 1988). Being male, young, and from a deprived socioeconomic background and having low intelligence or a history of substance abuse are clear risk factors.

Since violence is the result of a complex interaction of social, psychological, and biological antecedents, when assessing the potential for immediate danger, the interviewer will have to evaluate all of these specific areas and reach any conclusions carefully. Attention should be paid to one's personal feelings and the environment in which the patient is being screened. A careful evaluation is mandatory for all potentially aggressive patients.

REFERENCES

Beck, J.C., White, K.A., & Gage, B. (1991). Emergency psychiatric assessment of violence. *American Journal of Psychiatry, 148*, 1562–1565.

Haven, E., & Piscitello, V. (1989). The patient with violent behavior. In S.J. Lewis, R.K. Grainger, W.A. McDowell, R. Gregory, & R.L. Messner (Eds.), *Manual of psychosocial nursing interventions* (pp. 187–204). Philadelphia: Saunders.

James, D.V., Fineberg, N.A., Shah, A.K., & Priest, R. (1990). An increase in violence in an acute psychiatric ward: A study of associated factors. *British Journal of Psychiatry, 156*, 846–852.

Katz, P., & Kirkland, F. (1990). Violence and social structure on mental hospital wards. *Psychiatry, 53*, 262–277.

Lion, J.R. (1987). Clinical assessment of violent patients. In L.H. Roth (Ed.), *Clinical treatment of the violent person* (pp. 1–20). New York: Guilford.

Monahan, J. (1988). Risk assessment of violence among the mentally disordered: Generating useful knowledge. *International Journal of Law and Psychiatry, 11*, 249–257.

Rice, M.E., Harris, G.T., Varney, G.W., & Quinsey, V.L. (1989). *Violence in institutions: Understanding, prevention, and control*. Lewistown, NY: Hogrefe & Huber.

Smith, J.E., & Hucker, S.J. (1991). Violence. *Current Opinion in Psychiatry, 4*, 841–845.

5

Verbal Intervention

SUSAN LEWIS,
R.N., C.S., PH.D.

The prevention of physical violence is a major goal when working with angry, disturbed patients. In the majority of cases, verbal techniques are the primary mode of intervention. Used with empathy and respect, they can be very effective in defusing hostility and anger. Since violence rarely occurs suddenly and builds through a series of phases, the clinician often has the opportunity to use verbal intervention successfully; see Table 5-1. In general, patients are not randomly or irrationally violent, but react to significant stressors and situations (American Psychiatric Association, 1974).

Helplessness is the dynamic underlying aggression. Measures that assist the patient to feel less helpless and more in control can dissipate anger. Sometimes the acknowledgment of a person's angry feelings and the right to experience them can defuse a situation. In other instances, telling the patient in a calm, matter-of-fact manner, "We won't let you hurt yourself or anyone else," can reassure the individual that if there is a loss of control, the staff will intervene. In addition, this conveys that the staff *is* in control of the situation. Communication with the patient is crucial and should continue throughout the entire process even if physical restraint becomes necessary.

The psychiatric staff deals with patients' violent thoughts and verbalizations on a daily basis. The clinician's task is to assess the potential for violence and defuse it before physical assault occurs. Early intervention can significantly reduce the risk of attack. Most people in our society have not been taught to deal effectively with anger, either their own or that of others; therefore, acting-out patients are challenging and raise many emotions in those treating them. Therapists need education and training to cope with these various feelings and attitudes.

THE THREE ASPECTS OF SUCH SITUATIONS

In using verbal intervention, it is helpful to consider the situation from three aspects:

1. *Self.* What triggers me and what can I do about it? (Trimble & Van Fleet, 1988).
2. *Patient.* What circumstances have led to the patient's present condition?
3. *Environment.* What factors does the environment contribute to the patient's behavior, thoughts, and potential for violence?

Interventions that lessen the perceived threat and decrease feelings of impotence have the greatest potential for success (Rockwell, 1972).

Self

Every clinician is vulnerable at some point. The old adage "know thyself" is crucial in dealing with angry, hostile patients. The evaluator has to be aware of personal reactions to angry, violent people (Trimble & Van Fleet, 1988). An increase in muscle tension, palpitations, and diaphoresis are physical symptoms of perceived danger. The trigger may be verbal—sarcasm, racial slurs, or crude references to parentage. Words are potent triggers. Patients are adept at discovering the Achilles' heel.

Hostile or aggressive behavior on the part of the clinician can be a precipitant. At times a tendency to stereotype, prejudge, or feel personally attacked interferes with an objective, individually based evaluation.

Once the emotional response has been triggered, clinicians may be inclined to lash out and blame either the patient, themselves, or their co-workers. This hinders the ability to think logically and act effectively.

It is important to be aware of personal style and techniques when interviewing. Some professionals take a direct approach while others are less confrontative, respond more to feelings, and ask more questions. It is best to remain true to one's individual style; this is more likely to be perceived as sincere and genuine.

Victims can provoke violence through their attitude and approach to the patient. Sadness, anger, or frustration unrelated to the patient situation may contribute to the problem by making the therapist more irritable, impatient, and at risk of projecting personal feelings onto the patient.

Being aware of and controlling such personal feelings as anger and fear build confidence. Having a prearranged plan, having confidence in oneself and co-workers, and being adept at verbal skills will communicate competence and control.

Patient

As stated earlier, in most situations the primary dynamic motivating the angry patient is helplessness. The appropriate recognition of this need empowers the clinician and facilitates therapeutic intervention. Patients often use anger as a means of getting their needs met. In many cases, the system reinforces this behavior by reacting in some way to threats and intimidation or by giving in to demands.

Diagnosis is an important factor in predisposing a person to violence. This is discussed at length in Chapter 4. It is important to remember that (1) the more antisocial the behavior, the greater is the danger to staff, and (2) the presence of drugs or alcohol increases the risk considerably. Judgment is impaired and impulsivity is likely.

Environment

The setting can contribute significantly to violence; patients tend to live up to the expectations of the environment. If an angry, disruptive patient is thrust into a hostile or chaotic environment, disturbed behavior can escalate. Noise and confusion can heighten agitation. Crowding and inefficiency lead to frustration. The presence of an audience can incite and exacerbate a situation. Patients are quick to identify such problems as disorganization and staff conflict. Cohesiveness and team building are vital in decreasing environmental risk.

The environment should be designed to promote safety. A setting that communicates warmth and comfort is less harsh. Furniture and equipment should be chosen with security and protection in mind. Many items can be used by the patient as a weapon (e.g., letter openers, paperweights). The clinician can use other items as shields (e.g., light chair, cushion). It is preferable not to have sharp items or objects that can be thrown. An accessible panic button can alert others to danger and facilitate intervention and a quick response. Continuous observation is advised, as is awareness of the exits. Some hospitals have metal detectors similar to those used in airports.

When patients enter a health-care setting, they seek security and stability. The environment itself can effectively create a sense of emotional support and control.

INTERVENTION

A clinician who is alert to increasing tension can intervene before a situation erupts into violence. A number of basic, prudent measures can deter the attack.

Physically Approaching the Patient

Physical approach is the initial communication with the patient. Posture, facial expression, and tone of voice can be understood even by patients who cannot comprehend words when impaired by delirium, psychosis, anger, or fear (Parks, 1990). Facial expression should remain concerned, accepting, and attentive. When a patient is upset, the body buffer zone expands to four times that of one who is nonviolent. It is also greater to the rear than to the front (Parks, 1990). It is wise to approach the person at an angle slightly to the side as opposed to from behind (Figure 5-1). Facing a patient directly and entering the personal space can be perceived as confrontational. Do *not* touch this patient.

Although eye contact is influential, direct intense eye contact may be interpreted as a challenge. Stance is important; arms should not be folded in front, but should remain at the sides. In this position, they not only are less confrontational, but they are available to fend off a blow. Feet should be apart, one a little in front of the other, with the body at an angle. This allows better balance and makes the interviewer less of a target. Stand at least a leg's length away so that the patient would have to move in order to strike or grab.

One should *never* turn one's back on a disturbed patient. Make certain there is an accessible escape route. The area should be quiet and designed so that the individual can be observed continuously without feeling cornered or harassed. The staff members need to know where the interview is being conducted.

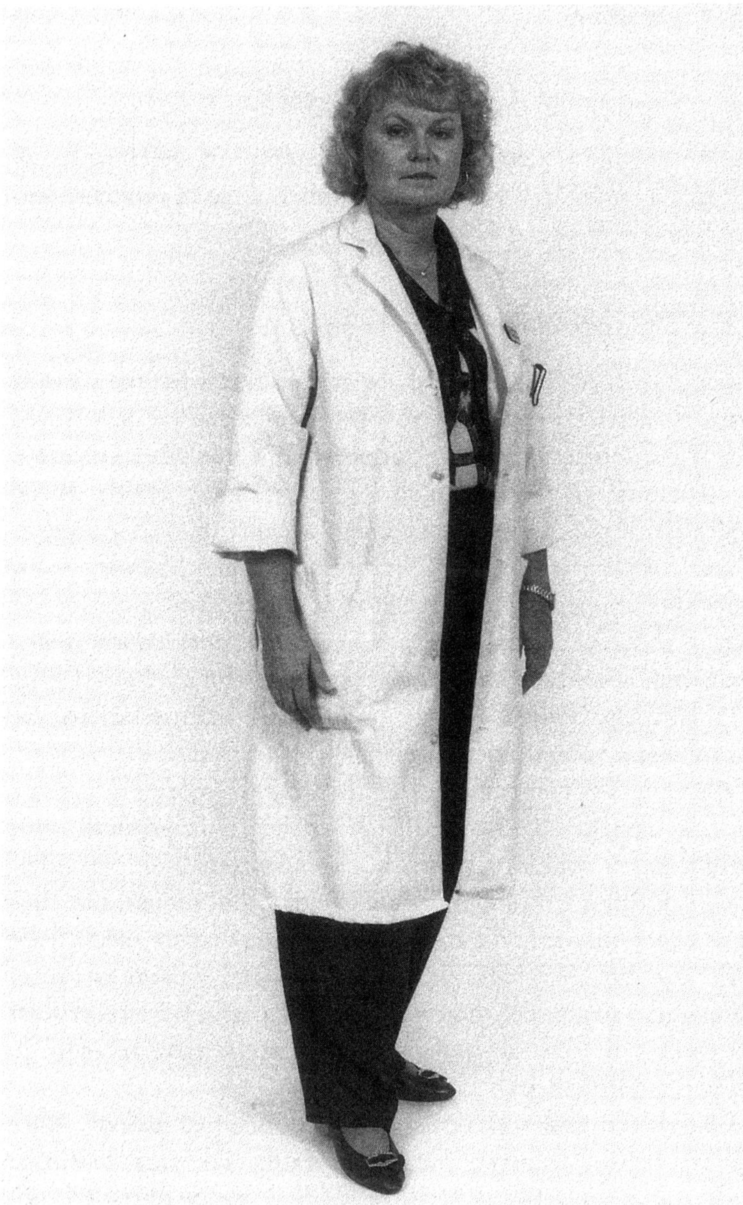

Figure 5-1 *(Photo Provided by Medical Media Service, Dept. of Veterans Affairs Medical Center, Louisville, Kentucky)*

Additional staff or security should stand by to help if necessary. Other patients and nonessential staff should be removed from the area.

Stay alert. Often a patient who intends to assault gives very little warning, striking very quickly. Although staring is not recommended, some eye contact is prudent. The patient will generally glance in the direction in which he or she plans to strike just prior to physical action.

Supportive Verbal Intervention

When supportive, empathic verbal skills are combined with active listening, most patients, even those who are psychotic, respond. Showing empathy does not mean that one agrees with the patient's reason or behavior, but indicates concern.

Be patient. Dealing with this type of patient requires time. The initial interview is not the appropriate time for attempts at interpretation and psychodynamic insight. It may provoke or start an argument. Comments and verbalizations should be simple and straightforward. It is safer not to alienate the angry person. It is recommended that one use surnames and appropriate titles (i.e., Mr., Ms., etc.) when addressing patients. This shows respect and establishes a professional atmosphere. The individual should be told the interviewer's name and position.

The level of hostility is assessed by noting the tone of voice, behavior, eyes, rude remarks, facial expression, limited attention span, and use of personal space. These are all clues to the patient's state of mind. It is useful to ascertain the individual's perception of the situation and the events that led up to the current crisis.

Patients can sense whether the clinician is genuine and honest and listens with empathy, calmness, and concern. The voice should be soft but firm. Do not belittle the patient. Do not argue. Body language and verbal content should be consistent.

It is futile to attempt to reason with somebody who is already out of control. In some cases, a command may be effective, "Stop! Put the chair down!"

Only promises that can be fulfilled should be made. Do not threaten or imply punishment. Threats are seen as a challenge. Punishment is the responsibility of the legal system. It is preferable to discuss consequences and appropriate choices and options. If someone else has better rapport with the patient, that person should assist. Offering food, beverages, or cigarettes is a warm gesture that can have a calming effect.

Threats by the patient to harm himself or herself or others should be taken seriously, reported to the appropriate source, and documented. When the staff knows there is an established course of action supported by the administration, the patient's actions are less upsetting.

Specific Techniques

See Trimble & Van Fleet, (1988)

1. *Ask questions.* This shows interest and concern. It helps to gain control and gives additional information. "When did you first suspect the CIA was monitoring your thoughts?" "What is the most violent thing you have ever done?"
2. *Disengage.* The patient is told that the clinician is leaving and why. This provides distance and allows time for the interviewer and the patient to calm down. "I am going to the nurses' station to check on your medication." When angry interactions are face-to-face with no relief in intensity, the interchange becomes more heated with an increasing rate of verbal exchange and level of hostility.
3. *Defer to a supervisor.* This can show that the patient is taken seriously. "I'm not able to handle your problem, but let me get my supervisor. She/he may be able to help you."

4. *Redirect the anger.* Redirecting the anger away from oneself can decrease the immediate risk. "The person you need to talk with is Dr X." It is also helpful to deflect the patient's anger from an individual to an institution.
5. *Identify a course of action and follow through.* "I would be angry too. Here's something you can do."
6. *Explore Options.* Give choices. This decreases helplessness. The choices may be limited, but they allow the patient to save face and feel in control. "Mr. X, I am running about an hour behind. Would you prefer to wait or would you like for me to reschedule you?" Or: *Patient:* "I'm going to report this to my senator!" *Clinician:* "Yes, that is an option. Let me give you his/her name and address."
7. *Demonstrate a helpful attitude.* "I am not sure that I can help you, but let me find out who can."

Setting Limits

Table 5-1 indicates various levels of rising tension and the appropriate intervention. If tension continues to mount, the patient will move from basic anxiety to threatening (Haven & Piscitello, 1989). This phase is characterized by such statements as: "Go to hell!" "You can't tell me what to do!" "I need my Xanax. If I don't get it this instant, someone will be very sorry!" Clenched fists and jaws and an angry tone of voice generally accompany threats.

Intervention at this level calls for continued verbal support with the addition of a directive, limit-setting component. Limit setting does not imply threatening the patient, but rather it involves setting appropriate limits to contain the situation (Haven & Piscitello, 1989). The key to successful limit setting is using only those limits that can be enforced. Once a limit is set, for example, "Let's go into my office and discuss this, the hallway

TABLE 5:1
Stage of Rising Tension and Appropriate Responses

Patient	*Staff*
I. Anxiety	I. Verbal intervention A. Assess what is occurring B. Use verbal techniques C. Attempt to calm the patient D. Do not invade the patient's personal space
II. Threatening	II. Setting limits A. Continue to use verbal techniques B. Set clear and definite limits C. Be directive and matter-of-fact D. Be prepared to enforce limits
III. Acting out	III. Team intervention—physical management skills A. Recognize mounting tension B. Designate a team leader C. Have a prearranged plan D. Function as a team E. Use only after other measures have failed
IV. Tension reduction	IV. Therapeutic rapport and emotional support A. Allow the patient to express his or her needs and feelings B. Listen nonjudgmentally C. Show concern for the patient D. Process the incident with other staff members without assigning blame

Adapted from Haven and Piscitello (1989).

is not the best place," and the patient says, "I'm not going anywhere with you!" the staff must be prepared either to escort a patient who is on the verge of acting out or to do nothing. Doing nothing is a sign that clinicians are helpless to assist in gaining control. This can be frightening to the patient, fostering further escalation and loss of control.

There are times when verbal intervention is not effective regardless of the clinician's skill. As threats approach acting out, physical intervention may become necessary. It is critical to use a team approach with a patient who is acting out. (see Chapter 7).

SUMMARY

Verbal techniques are basic in the prevention of violent behavior. Used with an empathic manner that conveys calmness, confidence, control, and a willingness to help, such techniques are extremely effective. Feelings of helplessness, fear of losing control, and/or psychosis are very painful and the patient wants relief. If the clinician can convey a genuine willingness to help, 85% to 90% of patients will respond to verbal intervention (Dubin, Benfield, & Berger, 1981).

REFERENCES

American Psychiatric Association (1974). *Clinical aspects of the violent individual.* Washington, D.C.: Author.

Dubin, W., Benfield, T., & Berger, M. (1981). Management of violent patients. Program excerpted from a symposium, *Management of Violent Patients in the Community* (pp. 3–10). New York: Pfizer Pharmaceuticals.

Haven, E., & Piscitello, V. (1989). The patient with violent behavior. In S. Lewis et al. (Eds.), *Manual of psychosocial nursing interventions* (pp. 187–204). Philadelphia: Saunders.

Parks, J. (1990). Violence. In J.R. Hillard (Ed.), *Manual of clinical emergency psychiatry* (pp. 147–160). Washington, D.C.: American Psychiatric Press.

Rockwell, D. (1972). Can you spot potential violence in a patient? *Hospital Physician, 10*, 52–56.

Trimble, D., & Van Fleet, F. (1988). Defusing hostility: Turning conflict into cooperation. Film produced by Uidatron Communications, Inc.

6

Pharmacotherapy of Violence

PATRICIA E. BLUMENREICH, M.D.

Aggression is a symptom, and as such, it is the result of multiple etiologies. It can be the consequence of a well-defined psychiatric or neurological illness or be of less clear origins. Psychotropic drugs are prescribed to treat the expressed violence and the underlying cause, if possible. There is no medication specifically intended for the treatment of aggressive behavior. Nevertheless, there are a number of pharmaceuticals that are employed to decrease or eliminate violence in either its acute or chronic manifestations. Drugs are generally not applied in circumstances of aggression related to criminality or personality disorders. This chapter focuses on guidelines for pharmacotherapy in a patient population.

ACUTE TREATMENT OF VIOLENCE

Antipsychotics

Description

Antipsychotic drugs or neuroleptics are medicines that were first developed to be used in anesthesia in the early 1950s. Their efficacy has been established for the treatment of psychotic conditions, such as in schizophrenia, mania, and other disorders.

Mechanism of Action

These agents block the postsynaptic dopamine receptors in selected pathways (Gelenberg, 1991). There are two major types of dopamine receptors, but no one drug is available that is specific to either one (Schatzberg & Cole, 1991). Their effectiveness in blocking the D_2 subtype of receptor correlates best with clinical potency (Gelenberg, 1991).

Indications

Neuroleptics are utilized to treat the symptoms of acute and/or chronic psychosis attributable to schizophrenia, mania, or other delusional disorders. Calming violence and agitated behavior is one of the principal therapeutic aims initially. They may also be applied in cases of psychoses arising from a dementia, delirium, or other organic brain syndrome.

Contraindications

Movement disorders such as Parkinson's disease or tardive dyskinesia are relative contraindications. The physician always must balance the benefits of using a medication against a worsening of the neurological function. Although a teratogenic effect of neuroleptics has not been demonstrated, it is safer to avoid them during pregnancy if possible, particularly during the first trimester.

Recommended Workup Prior to Treatment

Begin with a history and physical examination. Suggested laboratory evaluations include a hemogram, or complete blood count (CBC), and a serum chemistry survey to assess the general health status. In females, a negative human chorionic gonadotropin assay is often recommended to rule out a current pregnancy. An electrocardiogram is requested if cardiac disease is present or in people over 40 years of age.

Treatment

Antipsychotic drugs are used to diminish violence by treating the psychosis, regardless of etiology. They also tend to reduce agitation. Both low-dose, high-potency versions and high-dose, low-potency ones are effective. The pharmaceutical of choice often will be the one that has been most beneficial to the patient before.

The high-potency types are less sedative, have fewer anticholinergic or adrenolytic side effects, and may be safer in the elderly. Haloperidol, fluphenazine, and thiothixene are three such drugs. Haloperidol and fluphenazine also have the advantage of availability in a parenteral, extended-duration format (decanoate). Patients can be switched to a depot form of the medication after the symptoms are controlled. This is particularly beneficial for people with poor oral drug-taking compliance records.

The recommended doses of haloperidol are 3–5 mg intramuscularly (IM) or 5–10 mg orally (PO) every six hours or the equivalent. This quantity may suffice. In acutely psychotic, healthy persons with a significant risk of dangerous behavior, one may prescribe doses of 5–10 mg of haloperidol IM every two to four hours until sedation is achieved. With elderly or debilitated patients, the doses should be lower, in the range of 0.5–2 mg initially. Once the violent outburst is under control, 5–10 mg a day may be sufficient. The low-potency, higher-dose selections, such as chlorpromazine or thioridazine, are more sedative and induce fewer neurological, extrapyramidal side effects. The recommended doses range from 25 to 100 mg PO of chlorpromazine or its equivalent every one to four hours until sedation is achieved. In some severe cases, doses up to 800 mg of thioridazine or 1000 mg of chlorpromazine per day may be needed. Prescribed quantities are decreased to 200–600 mg a day when the violent episode has subsided. The amount of medicine administered generally is reduced as one passes from the phase of acute combativeness or agitation to a calm but still psychotic stage, and finally to one requiring a smaller maintenance, prophylactic quantity.

Clozapine, the newest antipsychotic, may offer symptom control to a number of previously treatment-resistant patients. To date, the impact of clozapine on violence secondary to psychosis has not been documented.

Side Effects

Antipsychotic medicines have a wide range of side effects and affect different systems during various stages of treatment. The following is a description of those manifestations.

Neuromuscular. Extrapyramidal side effects occur shortly after the initiation of treatment and usually within the first two or three weeks. They include acute dystonia, akathisia, and parkinsonism. They appear more frequently with the high-potency group. Dystonic reactions are characterized by sustained posturing of the neck, trunk, jaw, or eye musculature; protrusion of the tongue; or extreme upward gaze of the eyes. Relief can be quickly achieved with diphenhydramine 25–50 mg or benztropine 1–2 mg IM or intravenously (IV).

Akathisia is described as a restless inability to sit still or a need to pace about. It may be mistaken for an escalation of agitation and be treated erroneously with a higher neuroleptic dosage, with a subsequent worsening of symptoms. This very uncomfortable side effect can be treated with benztropine, trihexyphenidyl, propranolol, or a benzodiazepine, or by a reduction in the neuroleptic dose.

Parkinsonism is manifested by rigidity, masklike facies, slowness, and resting tremor. Benztropine 1–2 mg, trihexyphenidyl mg, amantadine 100 mg, or diphenhydramine 25 mg two to four times a day may be effective. Akinesia, a related symptom that is manifested by apathy and difficulties in initiating movement or speech, is treated like parkinsonism.

Sedation. This is a common side effect with low-potency, high-dose antipsychotics. It may be a desirable aspect in the very agitated, out-of-control patient. Tolerance to this manifestation may develop after a few days or weeks of treatment.

Neuroleptic malignant syndrome. This is a severe condition characterized by high fever, extreme muscular rigidity, fluctuating levels of arousal and orientation, diaphoresis, and instability of blood pressure. Laboratory findings include increased creatinine phosphokinase and leukocytosis. This syndrome develops over 24 to 48 hours. It may present months after exposure to neuroleptic medication. A rapid increase in the dose of a high-potency antipsychotic may increase the risks of developing this potentially fatal side effect. The treatment includes immediate discontinuation of the medication, hydration, and lowering of temperature. Dantrolene, amantadine, and bromocriptine have been used with various results. If neuroleptics need to be restarted, the low-potency ones might offer a questionable safer alternative. Reexposure to neuroleptics after a bout of resolved neuroleptic malignant syndrome frequently requires a neuroleptic-free period of several weeks duration.

Seizures. The low-potency neuroleptics increase the risk of having a convulsion more than do the high-dose versions. Ictal induction is uncommon and somewhat dose related.

Autonomic. These include orthostatic hypotension, tachycardia, dry mouth, blurred vision, inhibition of ejaculation, constipation, and urinary retention. They are more frequent with the low-potency antipsychotics. Elderly patients are more likely to exhibit these symptoms, and thus a high-potency drug is preferable for patients of that age group.

Cardiac. Prolonged QT interval and U-waves may appear on an electrocardiogram. Thioridazine may be the biggest offender in this regard.

Cutaneous. Patients on neuroleptics, especially chlorpromazine, may have an increased sensitivity to the sun and develop severe sunburns or rashes. Such persons should avoid the sun and wear sunscreen lotion if changes in the medication are not recommended.

Hormonal. Amenorrhea is commonly reported in maintenance-treated cases. Erratic menses, galactorrhea, gynecomastia in men, decreased libido, erectile dysfunction, and an inability to reach orgasm are all observed.

Hematologic. Agranulocytosis, though very rare, may occur within the first three months and can be fatal. Antipsychotics should be discontinued if neutropenia and infection are observed. A gradual, modest decrease in the white blood count is usually not serious and treatment can continue.

Ocular. Thioridazine in doses higher than 800 mg a day can produce pigmentary retinopathy. Corneal and lenticular depositions are also reported in neuroleptic-treated persons.

Drug Interactions

There is an increase in anticholinergic manifestations when neuroleptics are prescribed together with antiparkinsonian medications (i.e., benztropine). The sedative potential increases when administered with antihistamines (i.e., diphenhydramine), benzodiazepines (i.e., diazepam), or any sedative hypnotic, including alcohol. The possibility of respiratory depression and of a risk in operating dangerous machinery exist. When antipsychotics and cyclic antidepressant medicines are prescribed together, the blood levels of both increase. Severe neurotoxicity has been described in four patients receiving lithium and haloperidol (Gelenberg, 1991), but this reaction is rare and may be a form of neuroleptic malignant syndrome. Propranolol increases the blood levels of thioridazine and other neuroleptics (Tardiff, 1989). Antipsychotic drugs decrease the metabolism of phenytoin.

Anxiolytics

BENZODIAZEPINES

Description

Benzodiazepines (BZDs) are antianxiety agents and the most commonly prescribed psychotropic drugs. Examples include diazepam, chlordiazepoxide, and lorazepam (Rosenbaum & Gelenberg, 1991).

Mechanism of Action

Benzodiazepines block the stimulation that originates in the brain-stem reticular system and decrease the activity in areas associated with emotion, such as the hippocampus, hypothalamus, septal region, and amygdala. Their chemistry is not completely known. There are BZD receptors in the limbic system, cortex, and thalamic nuclei. The activity of the inhibitory neurotransmitter, gamma-aminobutyric acid, increases when the drug and the receptor interact.

Indications

Benzodiazepines are used as antianxiety agents, muscle relaxants, and hypnotics in preoperative anesthesia, status epilepticus, and alcohol withdrawal. They are the drugs of first choice to abort a violent episode when it is either imminent or occurring.

Benzodiazepines are not recommended for the long-term treatment of violence because of their potential for abuse, addiction, tolerance, sedation, and depression. In a study of normal subjects, the acute administration of diazepam decreased aggressivity; however, an increase in aggression was observed in some persons with relatively high hostility scores (Cherek, Steinberg, Kelly, Robinson, & Spiga, 1990). Parenteral administration of lorazepam is as effective as haloperidol in decreasing aggressive behavior and there is a greater decrease in the aggression ratings, independent of sedative effects (Salzman et al., 1991).

Contraindications

Caution should be used in pregnancy, particularly during the first trimester, because there have been reports of dysmorphogenesis. Benzodiazepines are not recommended for long-term use in individuals with alcohol and/or drug abuse histories because of their potential to be abused and their potentially dangerous addictive effects. There are reports of emotional dyscontrol with benzodiazepines (Dietch & Jennings, 1988).

Workup Prior to Use

Since BZD will be used in an emergency, there may not be enough time to obtain laboratory tests. Efforts should be made to obtain liver function and pregnancy tests and a toxicology screen as soon as possible.

Treatment

In emergencies, the short-acting drugs are often preferred. Since the IM route may be chosen, lorazepam is the most widely used. This drug is well absorbed PO, IM, and IV, and has no metabolites. It is safe to use it with other medicines. It is not absorbed into the tissues as rapidly as diazepam, it stays longer in the circulation, and it produces sedation for a longer period. Its half-life is 12 hours (diazepam's is 20–100, chlordiazepoxide's 5–30, and prazepam's 30–200) (Gelenberg, 1991).

The recommended dose of lorazepam is 1–4 mg PO or IM, repeated every two to four hours as needed, with a maximum of 12 mg in 24 hours. When given IV, it should be administered slowly, 2 mg (1 ml) per minute, and not more than 4 mg. This route should be used only in *very* severe cases.

Monitoring

The patients treated with these drugs have to be monitored for respiratory depression and laryngospasm. Resuscitation equipment must be readily available. Observe for instances of oversedation.

Side Effects

Benzodiazepines have a high therapeutic index and thus are very safe drugs. They produce sedation, which is a desirable effect when treating violence. Toxic doses produce decreased coordination and ataxia.

Drug Interactions

Alcohol may increase diazepam blood levels and it potentiates central nervous system (CNS) depressant effects. Diazepam increases phenytoin and digoxin concentrations. Disulfiram increases chlordiazepoxide and diazepam levels. Cimetidine increases the levels of long-acting BZD in the blood.

BARBITURATES

Description

Barbiturates are CNS depressants that today have a very limited use in psychiatry. They have been largely replaced by BZD.

Indications

Amobarbital may be used in psychiatric emergencies to induce sleep. It can be used as a calming agent, but BZDs are much safer and should generally obviate barbiturate use.

Contraindications

Barbiturates are contraindicated in patients with acute intermittent porphyria.

Workup Prior to Use

Liver function tests are recommended. Barbiturates are metabolized in the liver and a decrease in their metabolism may induce increased doses that may, in turn, end in a toxic state.

Treatment

Sodium amobarbital can be administered IV in a 10% aqueous solution. The recommended dose is 200–500 mg given not faster than 1 mg per minute (Tardiff, 1989).

Monitoring

Carefully monitor breathing to prevent respiratory depression and laryngospasm. Have resuscitation equipment readily available. Barbiturates have a low therapeutic index.

Drug Interactions

Barbiturates diminish anticoagulant action.

LONG-TERM TREATMENT OF VIOLENCE

Except for the antipsychotics, which are used for both the acute and chronic treatment of violence, all other medicines are restricted to use either in an emergency, such as the anxiolytics (except buspirone), or continuously, such as the mood stabilizers or anticonvulsants.

The long-term treatment of violence has to include other therapeutic modalities apart from medications. Individual and/or group psychotherapy, family counseling, Alcoholics Anonymous, and Narcotics Anonymous are some of the resources a therapist can use to improve the outcome.

Compliance with treatment is of paramount importance. Lack of improvement may point toward poor compliance and the doctor should always assess whether the medication is taken as prescribed and address this issue regularly.

Antipsychotics

Treatment

Maintenance treatment to prevent violence with neuroleptics is indicated in those persons whose aggressive behavior is secondary to psychosis of functional and organic bases. Haloperidol and fluphenazine are often used in their decanoate forms. The initial dose of haloperidol is 10–15 times the previous daily administration in haloperidol equivalents, but no more than 100 mg (2 ml). Monthly or biweekly injections are commonly recommended, but this schedule is adjusted to each individual's response and tolerance. Increments higher than 300 mg are usually not needed or advised. The starting dose of fluphenazine in its decanoate form is 25 mg (1 cc) every two to three weeks, usually not exceeding 100 mg every two to three weeks. It may be useful to start at 12.5 mg as a test dose, especially in older persons. If the low-potency, high-dose antipsychotic medicines are chosen for long-term pharmacotherapy, the doses will range from 200 to 800 mg of thioridazine or chlorpromazine a day, or its equivalent. People with anxiety and/or insomnia often prefer these agents because of their calming value.

Monitoring

There are no routine laboratory investigations that are essential or established as guidelines regarding the frequency of monitoring. A hemogram and liver enzyme tests are recommended each year. Clinically, patients should be checked at each visit, or a minimum of two to four times per year, for extrapyramidal (EPS) side effects and/or tardive dyskinesia. Documenting a formal Abnormal Involuntary Movement Scale (AIMS) assessment periodically can provide a standardized way to follow up evaluations.

Tardive dyskinesia is among the most feared long-term side effects of neuroleptics. It is characterized by involuntary choreoathetoid movements of the face, jaw, tongue, lips, extremities, and occasionally trunk. Wormlike movements of the tongue may be early-warning signs of its impending presence. Usually, drug exposure has lasted many months for this chronic ailment to develop. There is no convincing evidence that any one neuroleptic is less likely to induce tardive dyskinesia than others. Elderly patients, females, and individuals with mood disorders may be at greater risk. The symptoms may worsen after discontinuation of the drug. Some patients improve very gradually after a few months and others after a year or more. Bromocriptine and levodopa have been tried as alternative treatments if drug discontinuation is insufficient or clinically contraindicated. Benzodiazepines, such as diazepam, may be helpful. Prevention, by using the lowest effective dose, is the best advice.

Anxiolytics

BUSPIRONE

Description

Buspirone is a nonbenzodiazepine antianxiety agent that has been reported to be useful in the long-term treatment of aggression (Ratey, Sovner, Parks, & Rogentine, 1991). It has no place in acute care.

Mechanism of Action

Buspirone is a lipophilic compound that interacts with dopamine receptors, mainly presynaptic and the postsynaptic 5-HT1A (Rosenbaum & Gelenberg, 1991).

Indications

Buspirone has demonstrated effectiveness in the treatment of anxiety and aggression in the mentally retarded (Ratey et al., 1991). In this study, the decrease in aggression was independent of the antianxiety effect. There are no substantiated data regarding its usefulness in the non–mentally-retarded, violent population. It may be reasonable to try it.

Contraindications

There are no specific contraindications to its use. Although this drug does not increase the impairment caused by alcohol significantly, patients should be advised not to use them concomitantly.

Workup Prior to Use

A physical examination and baseline laboratory studies are recommended.

Treatment

Treatment can start at 5 mg three times a day and increase 5 mg every three days until a maximum dose of 40–60 mg is reached.

Monitoring and Side Effects

There have been no definitive extrapyramidal reactions attributed directly to buspirone at usual dosages, although there have been some reports associated with higher dosages. This drug seems unlikely to produce tardive dyskinesia.

Drug Interactions

Buspirone has no significant interaction with alcohol or other CNS depressants.

Anticonvulsants

CARBAMAZEPINE

Description

Carbamazepine was originally developed in 1957 for the treatment of epilepsy and other neuronal irritabity syndromes (e.g., tic douloureux). In the early 1970s, it began to be used to treat bipolar disorder refractory to lithium (Schatzberg & Cole, 1991). Currently, this agent is widely prescribed for the long-term prevention of impulsivity and emotional dyscontrol.

Biochemical Aspects

Carbamazepine is a dibenzazepine structurally related to tricyclic antidepressants.

Indications

Carbamazepine has been approved as an anticonvulsant to treat complex partial seizures and other types of convulsions of the clonic–tonic type. It is also effective in decreasing aggression due to conduct, personality, and/or organic disorders (Mattes, Rosenberg, & Mays, 1984). There is evidence of its efficacy in the treatment of bipolar patients when lithium is either ineffective or ill advised. It has been shown to be useful in decreasing impulsivity in borderline personality disorders (Cowdry & Gardner, 1988), in assaultiveness associated with frontal lobe dysfunction (Foster, Hillbrand, & Chi, 1989), and in the episodic violence of a case of multiple personality disorder (Fichtner, Kuhlman, Gruenfeld, & Hughes, 1990). It is also useful in treating the angry outbursts and poor impulse control of patients with combat-related post-traumatic stress disorder. This drug is not indicated for the acute treatment of violence.

Contraindications

Although it was believed until recently that this was the safest anticonvulsant to be employed in pregnancy, fetal abnormalities have been reported with its use (Schatzberg & Cole, 1991). Caution is advised when treating patients with brain damage or mental retardation because there have been reports of paradoxical worsening (Tardiff, 1989). Carbamazepine is contraindicated in patients with liver disease, bone marrow suppression, or tendencies toward hyponatremia.

Workup Prior to Use

Recommended laboratory testing includes a hemogram and hepatic function and electrolyte studies.

Treatment

Treatment may start with 100–200 mg at bedtime and the dosage increased by 200 mg daily to weekly or less often, based on the person's ability to tolerate its side effects. The average doses range from 400 to 1200 mg a day on a divided schedule. Results can be reported within the first few days to weeks of treatment.

Monitoring

Although there is little documented correlation between carbamazepine levels and the control of psychiatric symptoms, the drug blood levels are routinely monitored. They are checked 12 hours after the last dose. Values from 6 to 12 μg/ml are considered therapeutic. Once the desired response has been achieved at a steady-state level, assays are monitored once a month for three months, and every three to six months afterwards. A blood count and hepatic enzyme and electrolyte tests are monitored closely for the first three months, and three to six months after that.

Side Effects

The major concern is the appearance of agranulocytosis, thrombocytopenia, or a similar presentation of bone marrow suppression. Severe blood dyscrasias are rare and appear in only one out of 125,000 cases (Weilburg & Murray, 1991). Patients should be instructed to contact the physician if fever, sore throat, petechiae, bleeding, or bruising appears. Hematologic consultation should be sought. Mild leukopenia and anemia do occur during the first weeks of treatment. In management, for example, if the leukocyte count were down to $3000/mm^3$ with a normal differential and the patient seemed to benefit from the drug, it would not be necessary to discontinue carbamazepine. Close observation would then be mandated. Rashes have been reported in 5–15% of patients and sensitivity to the sun may be increased. When dermatologic disorders such as epidermal necrolysis, exfoliative dermatitis, and urticaria appear, the drug has to be discontinued. Side effects such as nausea, vertigo, sedation, and blurred vision may be reported at the onset of treatment and disappear with ongoing treatment. Since carbamazepine induces hepatic microsomal enzymes, it affects the blood levels of a variety of medications.

Drug Interactions

Carbamazepine interacts with numerous drugs. It decreases the effect of oral anticoagulants, corticosteroids, haloperidol, and valproic acid, and increases the toxicity of antidepressants and lithium.

There is an increase in carbamazepine's toxicity when cimetidine is added.

Noradrenergic Agents

Description

Beta-blockers are drugs approved by the U.S. Food and Drug Administration (FDA) for the treatment of hypertension and in the prophylaxis of angina, arrhythmias, and migraine headaches.

Biochemical Aspects

These agents block beta nor-adrenergic receptors in the peripheral sympathetic system and possibly also at a central level.

Uses

Apart from the above-mentioned uses, beta-blockers are used in psychiatry for the treatment of akathisia and anxiety. Several studies have demonstrated their usefulness to control violence in patients with many types of organic brain disease, mental retardation, dementia, and Huntington's, Wilson's, or Korsakoff's disease. They are not indicated in the acute treatment of violence (Silver & Yudofsky, 1985; Ruedrich, Grush, & Wilson, 1990; Luchins & Dojka, 1989). Alpha-blockers, such as clonidine, have calming effects too, and have been used in some cases.

Contraindications

Beta-blockers are contraindicated in varying degrees for persons with asthma, chronic obstructive pulmonary disease, congestive heart failure, diabetes mellitus, severe renal disease, hyperthyroidism, or depression.

Workup Prior to Use

A blood pressure measurement, a glycemia test, and an electrocardiogram are recommended.

Treatment

In order to treat violence with propranolol, it is advisable to start at 10–20 mg a day. Evaluate for hypotension and bradycardia, and if well tolerated, propranolol can be increased to 20 mg three times a day and increased by 20–60 mg every four days. Propranolol should be reduced if the pulse drops below 50 beats per minute or the systolic pressure is 90 or less. The same applies if dizziness, wheezing, or ataxia occurs. Doses above 600–800 mg a day are rarely needed. Nadolol, pindolol, and metoprolol have also been reported to be effective in some cases (Silver & Yudofsky, 1985). A drug trial of eight weeks at the maximun tolerated dose is recommended before calling the treatment a failure. If discontinuation is needed, propranolol should be decreased by 60 mg every day until 60 mg is reached. Then it is decreased by 20 mg every other day. Sudden discontinuation may trigger rebound severe hypertension. Depression has been reported as a side effect of propranolol.

Drug Interactions

Propranolol may increase blood levels of neuroleptics, particularly thioridazine. Beta-blockers delay recovery from insulin-induced hypoglycemia. Propranolol enhances the pressor response to epinephrine.

Psychostimulants

Description

Psychostimulants are sympathomimetics used mainly in the treatment of childhood attention-deficit disorder (ADD) with hyperactivity.

Biochemical Aspects

Psychostimulants prevent catecholamine reuptake and their degradation by monoaminoxidase. They may have direct agonist activity.

Indications

They are used by experts in the field to treat children and adolescents who are violent as a consequence of ADD (Hinshaw, Buhrmester, & Heller, 1989; Barkley, McMurray, Edelbrock, & Robbins, 1989). They are used in long-term treatment only (Brizer, 1988).

Contraindications

Psychostimulants are contraindicated in people with anxiety, who are drug users, who exhibit psychosis, and those who are at risk of developing a tic disorder.

Workup Prior to Use

Liver function studies prior to use are always recommended.

Treatment

For dextroamphetamine, treatment is 5–40 mg per day. For magnesium pemoline, it is 1–2.5 mg/kg daily. For methylphenidate, it is 37.5–75 mg daily.

Monitoring

Growth should be monitored in children who are treated with these drugs for prolonged periods.

Side Effects

The following symptoms can develop with chronic use: insomnia, appetite suppression, psychosis, rebound symptoms with abrupt discontinuation, and decreased growth. Pemoline can alter liver function. Children with a family history of tics are at greater risk for developing a persistent tic disorder. Either a drug holiday or the use of another medication is indicated if side effects are too deleterious.

Drug Interactions

Stimulants may decrease the effect of certain hypertensive agents. They inhibit the metabolism of antidepressants, anticoagulants, and anticonvulsants. It is necessary to monitor blood levels when these drugs are coprescribed.

Lithium

Description

Lithium is a naturally occurring ion that, in its salt format, has been used to treat different conditions since the 1800s. Today, lithium carbonate is the preparation of choice.

Mechanism of Action

Lithium's mechanism of action is unclear. Different theories have been postulated: the correction of an ion-exchange abnormality; increases in the reuptake and metabolism of norepinephrine; a decrease of the availability of acetylcholine; an alteration of serotonin receptor sensitivity; an increase in the release of norepinephrine, serotonin, and dopamine; or an alteration of adenylate cyclase and membrane permeability (Gelenberg & Schoonover, 1991).

Indications

Lithium is used to treat hypomania, mania, and recurrent or chronic affective disorders, and to enhance the efficacy of antidepressants. It is also used to treat poor impulse control, aggressive behavior, children with conduct disorder or hyperactivity, and organic brain syndromes. Lithium has proved to be useful in the treatment of violent, nonpsychotic prison inmates (Sheard, 1971; Sheard, Marini, Bridges, & Wagner, 1976).

Workup Prior to Use

Lithium can affect many organs; therefore, a complete medical examination and laboratory tests have to be done prior to its use. The history will focus on symptoms or illnesses that affect the kidneys (i.e., diabetes mellitus, hypertension), the thyroid, the parathyroid (i.e., hyperparathyroidism), and the cardiac system. Required laboratory tests are tests of thyroid function, thyroid-stimulating hormone (TSH), and serum calcium; an electrocardiogram, if over 40 years old; a hemogram; a pregnancy test; a urine analysis; and tests of fasting blood sugar, blood urea nitrogen (BUN), serum creatinine, creatinine clearance, and electrolytes.

Treatment

Lithium levels to control aggression should be in the range of 0.5–1.2 mEq per liter. Doses can range from 450 to 2100 mg/day based on clinical and laboratory parameters.

Monitoring

The lithium level should be obtained a few days after the first day of treatment, at 12 hours after the last dose. After a few weeks and once a desired level has been reached, check levels monthly for the first six months and every three to five months afterwards. A CBC can be checked once a year.

Thyroid tests (T_3,T_4,TSH) should be obtained every six months afterwards, likewise for fasting glucose and serum creatinine.

Contraindications

Lithium is absolutely contraindicated in pregnancy, particularly during the first trimester due to the possibility of cardiac malformations. People with seizure disorders or electroencephalogram abnormalities might constitute relative contraindications.

Side Effects

When the level is low or therapeutic, common side effects include nausea, diarrhea, tremor, malaise, and fatigue. The gastric irritation can be treated by taking lithium after meals, decreasing the dose, using a sustained-release preparation, or further dividing the dose. Propranolol can be useful in treating lithium-induced tremor. Long-term side effects include a decrease in the kidneys' maximal concentrating capacity (such as nephrogenic diabetes insipidus). Glomerular filtration is minimally impaired. Adequate fluid intake (as much as necessary to remain hydrated), a diet low in protein and solutes, diuretics, and a once-a-day schedule for lithium are useful to decrease polyuria (Gelenberg & Schoonover, 1991).

Adverse cardiac reactions are rare. Lithium can worsen skin disorders such as psoriasis. Weight gain is common. At the CNS level, it can decrease memory and concentration, and patients may complain of fatigue, headache, and lethargy. Lithium can cause a clinically significant hypothyroidism and a diffuse non-tender goiter. These disorders remit if the lithium is discontinued.

At toxic levels, lithium can produce ataxia, lethargy, dizziness, slurred speech, nystagmus, nausea, and vomiting. When the blood level is above 2 mEq per liter, symptoms also may include severe blurred vision, fasciculations, clonic movements of the body, hyperactive reflexes, choreoathetoid movements, electroencephalogram changes, toxic psychosis, syncope, circulatory failure, and coma. If such symptoms persist or worsen, convulsions, oliguria, permanent cerebellar injury, and/or death can follow.

Drug Interactions

The following are some of the drugs that can affect lithium levels.

These drugs can increase lithium levels: thiazide diuretics, triamtirene, spironolactone, phenylbutazone, indomethacin, ibuprofen, angiotensin converting enzyme (ACE) inhibitors. These drugs can decrease lithium levels: caffeine, theophylline, osmotic diuretics. Toxic symptoms with normal blood levels can appear with methyldopa and cardiovascular toxicity with hydroxyzine.

CONCLUSION

Aggression is a complex behavior and the result of multiple etiologies. Clinicians should maximize their efforts in trying to find an underlying psychiatric–medical disorder in the violent patient that could be successfully treated. Although there is no specific drug for the treatment of aggression, knowledge and expertise with various drug groups are needed to eliminate this dangerous behavior.

REFERENCES

Barkley, R.A., McMurray, M.B., Edelbrock, C.S., & Robbins, K. (1989). The response of aggressive and nonaggressive ADHD children to two doses of methylphenidate. *Journal of the American Academy of Child and Adolescent Psychiatry, 28*(6), 873–881.

Brizer, D.A. (1988). Psychopharmacology and the management of violent patients. *Psychiatric Clinics of North America, 11*(4), 551–569.

Cherek, D.R., Steinberg, J. L., Kelly, T. H., Robinson, D. E., & Spiga, R. (1990). Effects of acute administration of diazepam and d-amphetamine on aggressive and escape responding of normal male subjects. *Psychopharmacology, 100*(2), 173–181.

Cowdry, R., & Gardner, D. (1988). Pharmacotherapy of borderline personality disorder: Alprazolam, carbamazepine, trifluoperazine and tranylcypromine. *Archives of General Psychiatry, 45*, 111–119.

Dietch, J.T., & Jennings, R.K. (1988). Aggressive dyscontrol in inpatients treated with benzodiazepines. *Journal of Clinical Psychiatry, 49*, 184–188.

Fichtner, C.G., Kuhlman, D.T., Gruenfeld, M.J., & Hughes, J.R. (1990). Decreased episodic violence and increased control of dissociation in a carbamazepine treated case of multiple personality. *Biological Psychiatry, 27*, 1045–1052.

Foster, H.G., Hillbrand, M., & Chi, C.C. (1989). Efficacy of carbamazepine in assaultive patients with frontal lobe dysfunction. *Progress in Neuropsychopharmacology and Biological Psychiatry, 13*, 865–874.

Gelenberg, A. J. (1991). Psychoses. In A.J. Gelenberg, E.L. Bassuk, & S.C. Schoonover (Eds.), *The practitioner's guide to psychoactive drugs* (pp. 125–176). New York: Plenum.

Gelenberg, A. J., & Schoonover, S. C. (1991). Bipolar disorders. In A.J. Gelenberg, E.L. Bassuk, & S.C. Schoonover (Eds.), *The practitioner's guide to psychoactive drugs* (pp. 91–121). New York: Plenum.

Hinshaw, S.P., Buhrmester, D., & Heller, T. (1989). Anger control in response to verbal provocation: Effects of stimulant medication for boys with ADHD. *Journal of Abnormal Child Psychology, 17*(4), 393–407.

Luchins, D.J., & Dojka, D. (1989). Lithium and propranolol in aggression and self-injurious behavior in the mentally retarded. *Psychopharmacology Bulletin, 25*(3), 372–375.

Mattes, J.A., Rosenberg, J., & Mays, D. (1984). Carbamazepine versus propranolol in patients with uncontrolled rage outbursts: A random assignment study. *Psychopharmacology Bulletin*, *20*, 98–100.

Ratey J., Sovner R., Parks, A., & Rogentine, K. (1991). Buspirone treatment of aggression and anxiety in mentally retarded patients: A multiple-baseline, placebo lead-in study. *Journal of Clinical Psychiatry*, *52*(4), 159–162.

Rosenbaum, J.F., & Gelenberg, A.J. (1991). Anxiety. In A.J. Gelenberg, E.L. Bassuk, & S.C. Schoonover (Eds.), *The practitioner's guide to psychoactive drugs* (pp. 179–218) New York: Plenum.

Ruedrich, S.L., Grush, L., & Wilson, J. (1990). Beta-adrenergic blocking medications for aggressive or self-injurious mentally retarded persons. *American Journal on Mental Retardation*, *95*(1), 110–119.

Salzman C., Soloman D., Miyawaki, E., Glassman, R., Rood, L., Flowers, E., & Thayer, S. (1991). Parenteral lorazepam versus parenteral haloperidol for the control of psychotic disruptive behavior. *Journal of Clinical Psychiatry*, *52*(4), 177–180.

Schatzberg, A. F., & Cole, J. O. (1991). Antipsychotics. In A.F. Schatzberg & J.O. Cole, *Manual of clinical psychopharmacology.* Washington D.C.: American Psychiatric Press.

Sheard, M.H. (1971). Effect of lithium on human aggression. *Nature*, *230*, 113–114.

Sheard, M.H., Marini, J.L., Bridges, C.I., & Wagner, E. (1976). The effect of lithium on impulsive aggressive behavior in man. *American Journal of Psychiatry*, *133*(12) 1409–1413.

Silver, J.M., & Yudofsky, S. (1985). Propranolol for aggression: Literature review and clinical guidelines. *International Drug Newsletter*, *20*, 9–12.

Tardiff, K. (1989). Use of emergency medication. In K. Tardiff, *Assessment and management of violent patients.* Washington, D.C.: American Psychiatric Press.

Weilburg, J.B., & Murray, G.B. (1991). Temporolimbic epilepsy. In A.J. Gelenberg, E.L. Bassuk, & S.C. Schoonover (Eds.), *The practitioner's guide to psychoactive drugs* (pp. 407–437). New York: Plenum.

7

Physical Techniques

JAMES M. MORRISON, M.S.S.W.

This chapter centers on the physical techniques and principles used in the management of disruptive behavior, although prevention is always the primary consideration. No matter how skilled, well trained, or experienced a person is in the techniques of physical intervention, any type of bodily contact increases the risk of harm to both the staff member and the patient. Although training and expertise are important for the successful resolution of any physical conflict, they do not ensure personal safety. The first mandate for any health-care facility is to secure the personal health and safety of the patients and the staff. Therefore, verbal intervention, as mentioned in Chapter 5, is of great relevance to prevent further acting out. Self-protection through the use of physical defense mechanisms is only a last resort, once all other alternatives have been exhausted, the threat of physical attack is imminent, or physical contact has been initiated by either the patient or the staff.

The physical techniques detailed here are derived from the martial arts, but are primarily defensive in nature (Veterans Administration, 1987). They rely on the principles of speed, surprise, and leverage. The absence of any of these principles will affect the release mechanisms. For example, if you tell an individual to grab you in a hold to allow you to demonstrate a release

---

The photo illustrations in this chapter were provided by Medical Media Service, Dept. of Veterans Affairs Medical Center, Louisville, Kentucky.

technique, the element of surprise has been removed, resulting in a tighter grip and more difficulty in effecting a release. The described methods attempt to protect the staff members and the patient from harm to self or others without using force or pain.

The physical techniques and principles are divided into two major groups: personal safety skills and team skills. Personal safety skills are subdivided into preparatory techniques, grabs, and strikes and kicks. The use of weapons is also discussed.

PERSONAL SAFETY SKILLS

Personal safety skills are those release mechanisms based on a one-to-one confrontation in which a patient may grab, strike, or kick another person. The physical release techniques and principles deal with two different concepts: release and control versus release and escape. Release and control teach that once a hold has been released, the staff member will attempt to control the patient physically until assistance arrives or the patient has gained more self-control. The release-and-escape viewpoint states that once a physical hold release has been effected, as much physical space as possible will be placed between the patient and the staff member, while still providing for the safety of the patient. One-on-one situations can result in an increased risk of harm to both the patient and staff. Generally, release and physical distancing to increase personal space are desirable. Preparatory techniques include personal space, physical stance, eye contact, and falls.

Preparatory Techniques

Personal Space

Personal space is an invisible area that surrounds each individual and serves as a protective security zone. The distance or extent of that space will change according to the situation, individual mood, and the person or persons encroaching on that space. People are allowed within that personal space until the level of discomfort becomes too intense. When an agitated person is approached, make sure that the personal space is not violated. The presence of fear, anger, and other associated emotions can result in the personal space being much expanded. The patient should be approached no closer than a leg's length (that length should be equal to the longest leg—the staff member's or the patient's). The physical space will increase according to any escalation in the patient's behavior.

Physical Stance

Approach the patient in a nonadversarial way. The physical stance should be nonconfronting with one foot forward toward the patient and the other foot a half a step back at a 45-degree angle. Feet should be a distance apart that is equal to the width of the shoulders. This will place the body slightly toward the side that presents a less confrontational appearance while simultaneously giving the ability to move quickly forward or backward. Legs should be slightly flexed at the knees, not rigid or locked, in order to allow the shifting of weight.

This stance also provides a firm foundation against being pushed or pulled. Arms should be at the side, and never crossed, behind the back, or with the hands in the pockets.

Eye Contact

Eye contact with the patient is extremely important. It denotes care, concern, and involvement. Eye contact should be a casual observation, not a fixed stare. A stare only communicates challenge. Eye contact also gives advance warning of the delivery and target of strikes, grabs, or kicks. A blow will be preceded by a glance to that area. This allows some preparation for defense.

Just prior to the delivery of an overhead or downward blow, the attacker will quickly glance upward. A kick will be indicated by a downward glimpse.

Those trained and experienced in the martial arts are an exception to this rule. They will not disclose their moves in advance. Anyone trained in the martial arts should be treated as if armed with a weapon and handled by police officers or security personnel. Give them a large personal space.

Falls

Knowing how to fall is important to prevent injury. If pushed or shoved, one should relax and allow oneself to fall. This is actually very difficult, because falling creates a sense of lack of control. It is almost instinctual to stagger backwards while attempting to regain one's balance, which often results in a greater injury when one finally falls.

When coming down, take one step backward while bending at the hips. This allows the center of gravity to lower, thus reducing the chance of injury. The arms should be stretched outward. Allow the body to go down and back, landing on the buttocks and rolling onto the back. Simultaneously extend the arms at a 90-degree angle to the midline of the trunk and hit the floor with open palms to help absorb the force of the fall. The head should be held forward toward the chest. Do *not* attempt to break the force of the fall with the elbows. When on the floor, continue the defensive reaction by raising one leg, with the foot of that leg extended outward toward the patient. Rotate the trunk as the patient goes from side to side to keep the extended leg toward the attacker. Meanwhile, continue to use verbal skills until assistance arrives.

Grabs

Grabs will be discussed in the following order:

- Single grip on one arm
- Single grip on both arms
- Double grip on one arm (thumbs in the same direction)
- Double grip on one arm (thumbs in the opposite direction)
- Grasp of one elbow from behind
- Grasp of both elbows from behind
- Front strangle
- Rear strangle
- Front hair pull (one hand, both hands)
- Rear hair pull (one hand, both hands)
- Bear hug (front and rear)
- Grasp of tie, blouse, or shirt collar
- Bite
- Forearm choke
- Half nelson

As the grips and grabs are discussed, other releases that use similar tactics (i.e., breaking the grip at the weakest point and the use of surprise, speed, and leverage) are presented. Any release should be kept as simple as possible to avoid failure. Always run away from the patient after a release has been effected. Maintaining close proximity invites further attack.

Grips

A wrist or forearm gripped by one hand of a patient is defined as a "single" grip (see Figure 7-1). The weak part of the grasp is between the thumb and fingers. The release is initiated by taking one step toward the patient while shifting the weight toward that foot. Form the hand of the gripped arm into a fist. Twist the arm toward the gripping thumb until the side of the wrist

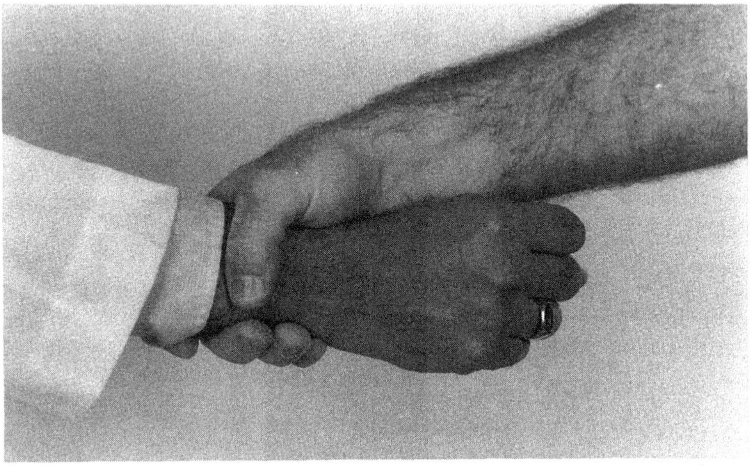

Figure 7-1

slips between the thumb and fingers (Figure 7-2). The entire strength of the arm and shoulder is used against one thumb. Step back with the leading foot while shifting the weight to that foot. Back away from the patient while continuing to use verbal skills. The free hand may be used to block the patient's free hand or to seize the patient's holding hand while the gripped hand is freed by the above method.

Both wrists or forearms may be clasped also. For the release, take one step toward the patient, shifting the weight onto that leg. Twist both wrists toward the thumbs of each of the gripping hands while pulling up and outward, thus releasing both wrists at the same time (same release as in the single wrist). Step away from the patient, shifting the weight onto the back leg.

A patient may grab one arm with both hands in the "double grip" (thumbs in the same direction), often from the side. Take one step toward the patient, shifting the weight onto the forward foot. Grasp the fist of the captured arm with the free hand and begin to push upward with the captured arm. When the coun-

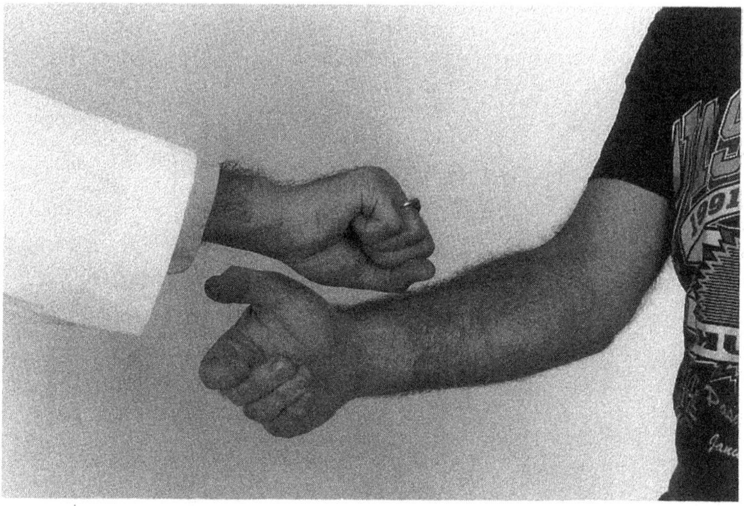

Figure 7-2

terpressure from the patient's grab is felt, push the captured arm downward abruptly, twisting it toward the thumbs of the patient. This will effect the release at the weak part of the grip between the thumbs and fingers. Shift weight toward the rear foot and step away from the patient (Figure 7-3).

The double grip on one arm (thumbs in the opposite direction) usually occurs from a frontal approach. Take one step toward the patient, shifting weight onto the forward foot. Form the hand of the captured arm into a fist. Grasp the hand of the captured arm with the free hand, reaching between the arms of the patient (Figure 7-4). Shift weight to the rear foot while pulling the captured hand and arm up and to the side, away from the captured arm. Continue to turn to the side, away from the captured arm, completing a full arc with the arms now released. Once in this position, step away or run. An elbow grasped from behind in a U-shaped grip is also a grab with its weak point at the junction of the thumb and fingers. Take one step ahead and make a sharp forward and upward movement with the captured arm. Yell for

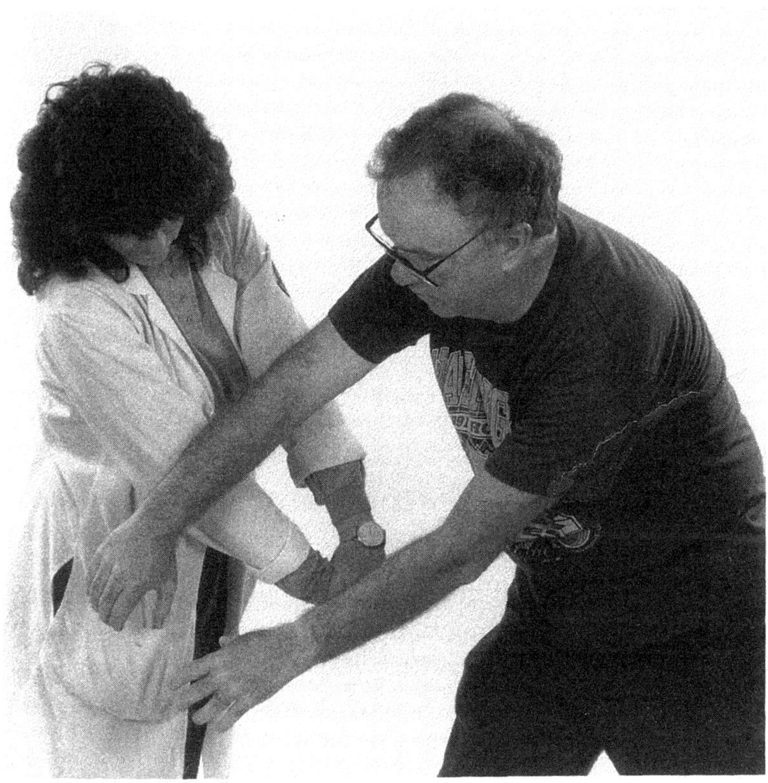

Figure 7-3

assistance and create a physical distance. If both elbows are grabbed from behind, the same procedures as above are used—just move both arms in the forward and upward movement simultaneously.

Strangles

The throat of a staff member gripped by both hands of an attacker is called a front strangle and is both dangerous and frightening. Quickly raise both arms into the air parallel to the midline of the body. Turn sharply to either side until facing completely away

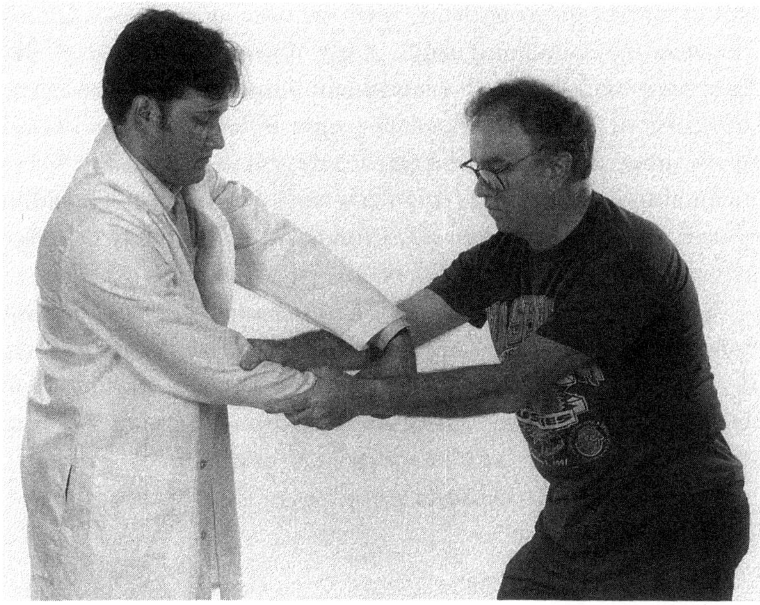

Figure 7-4

from the patient. This is the same mechanism as for breaking a grip at the junction of the fingers and thumbs using the leverage of the upper arms and shoulders. This technique facilitates escape from the patient. Run, creating distance from the attacker. The old methods of breaking this grab by sharply hitting the wrists of the attacker or reaching the arms upward through and between the arms of the assailant are rarely effective.

The rear strangle hold uses the same techniques as the front strangle, but ends facing the patient. It is especially important to step away so as not to remain within reach.

Hair Pulls

Hair pulls can be extremely painful and restraining. To release a front hair pull (one hand gripping the hair), place both hands on top of the capturing hand, with the edge of the hands against the wrist of the grabbing hand. Apply downward pressure on that hand with both hands. It is extremely important that the downward pressure be maintained as weight relieves the pain created by the grasp and applies leverage for the release of the hold. While maintaining the pressure, step back with one foot while bending quickly downward at the waist (Figure 7-5). Care must be taken to bend far enough in order to release the hold.

A front hair pull (two hands gripping) uses this same release, but each hand will be placed on top of each of the gripping hands. If possible, interlock the fingers of both hands to provide more leverage and pressure. Maintain the pressure against the head to effect the release and to control the pain.

A rear hair pull (one hand gripping) uses a similar technique.

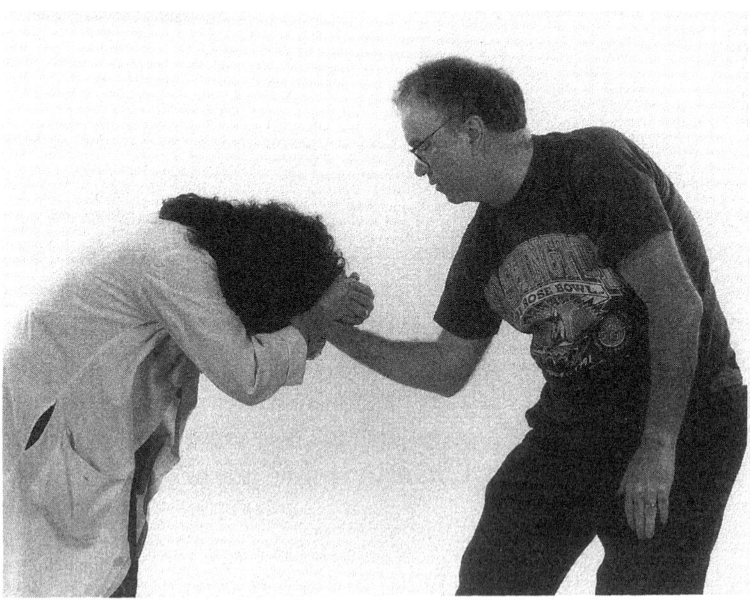

Figure 7-5

Place both hands on top of the capturing hand at the wrist. Put downward pressure on the capturing hand against the head to control the pain and to exert leverage. While maintaining pressure, rotate the body down and in toward the attacker until the body is toward him or her but the upper torso is parallel with the floor. While maintaining pressure, raise the upper torso into a standing position. This will bring the individual to his or her toes and effect release of the hold. At this point, release the hold to avoid injury to the patient.

A rear hair pull (two hands gripping) uses the same method as the rear hair pull with one hand gripping. The only difference in the release is that one hand is placed on top of each of the capturing hands. Interlock the fingers of both hands while keeping the edge of each palm against the wrist joint of the capturing hands.

Bear Hug

In a bear hug, the staff member faces the patient, and the normal reaction is to struggle while attempting to back away from the hold. Instead, embrace the attacker. Step with one leg to the outside and slightly forward. Either leg can be used as long as the leg steps to the same side—right leg to right side or left leg to left side. Immediately place the inner leg directly behind the legs of the patient to the same side and bend the person, with that leg acting as a fulcrum. Lay the patient on the ground very gently.

In a rear bear hug, do the same as above except that an embrace cannot be used in return. Instead, hold the patient's arms as tightly as possible and repeat the above steps.

Grasp of Clothes

On occasion, a patient may grab a tie, shirt front, or blouse in a threatening manner. Reach across the front of the chest with the arm on the thumb side of the grasping hand. Insert the fingers across the back of the grasping hand and into the palm. Rotate the clasping hand away from the grasp while using the free arm and hand to support the release by pushing the patient's shoulder.

Bites

A bite is both painful and dangerous. Avoid the almost instantaneous reaction of leaning back and pulling the affected limb away from the pain. That action will result in increased pain and physical injury. Instead, push in toward the bite. This reduces the pain and pressure of the bite through counterpressure. Be careful not to apply too much weight in order to avoid injury to the patient. Use the free hand to place the index finger into the pressure point just below the ear at the upper point of the mandible. Extend the thumb of the same hand to the lower frontal point of the mandible. Complete a jaw thrust and remove the injured area.

Chokes

A forearm choke is the most dangerous hold. A patient's forearm is placed around a staff member's neck from behind, while the other arm secures the hand of the choking arm. The attacker leans onto the victim and lifts his or her body off the ground. In addition to a decrease in the air supply, this hold can very easily break the victim's neck with any sudden move. This is the *only* technique in which inflicting pain is allowed. Sometimes, not even pain is sufficient. Turn and tuck the chin as much as possible into the V created by the elbow joint of the choking arm of the patient. This may improve breathing. With the side of a shoe, scrape the front of the attacker's leg from the knee to the instep of his or her foot, stomping hard onto the instep.

Since sudden pain may temporarily release some of the pressure of the choke, apply upper pressure at the V of the choking arm with the hand on the same side of the choking arm. At the same time, use the other hand to grab one to two fingers of the choking hand and apply outward pressure. Slip a hand through the area of the choking arm. As much physical distance as possible immediately should be put between the patient and victim. Whenever pain is inflicted, it may be reciprocated.

Half Nelson

In this hold, one arm is twisted behind the back and upward pressure is applied. This is painful, but in technical terms it is not a hold unless it is secured by a forearm choke, for example, even though it does produce discomfort. Simply step forward and turn away from the hold while straightening the arm, and the hold will be released.

Strikes and Kicks

Blocking is extremely important since it prevents strikes and blows from doing any damage, and gives some maneuverability to the staff member. A block consists of crossing both arms at the wrists to form a V. Hands are formed into fists to protect the fingers. The next phase of the block is to step into the kick or strike before the blow can reach its full force and extension. The block is swept either up or down depending on whether a strike or kick is being utilized (Figure 7-6). During the block, extend the arms and keep the eyes open to avoid injury. If the block is missed by the V of the hands, the strike or kick still can be deflected by the outer arms.

The block has to be successful before any other action can be used. Block and escape if nobody is available to help. After suc-

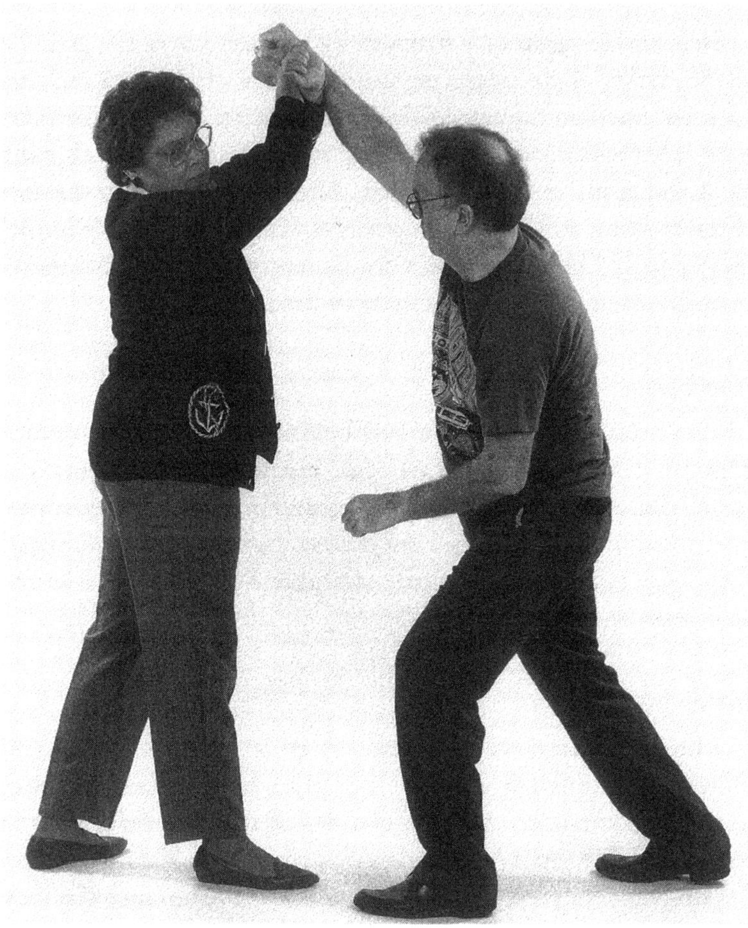

Figure 7-6

cessfully blocking a kick, it is possible to grab the leg at the point of contact and apply slight upward pressure to throw the patient off balance. However, this can easily lead to injury and should be avoided if possible.

In addition to the releases that have been summarized, many other techniques exist. Some of them use additional pressure points, leverage of fingers by bending them backward, and maneuvers that utilize more active force. Although these can be used as a last recourse, they are not encouraged because of their potential for injury to the patient.

A preferred block in response to a kick is a simple twisting of one leg to the side from the hip level (Figure 7-7). This will protect the groin area from injury, although it does leave the thigh area more vulnerable to receive the full force of the kick. Nevertheless, the staff member is still able to respond and the patient will not be injured as a result of this block.

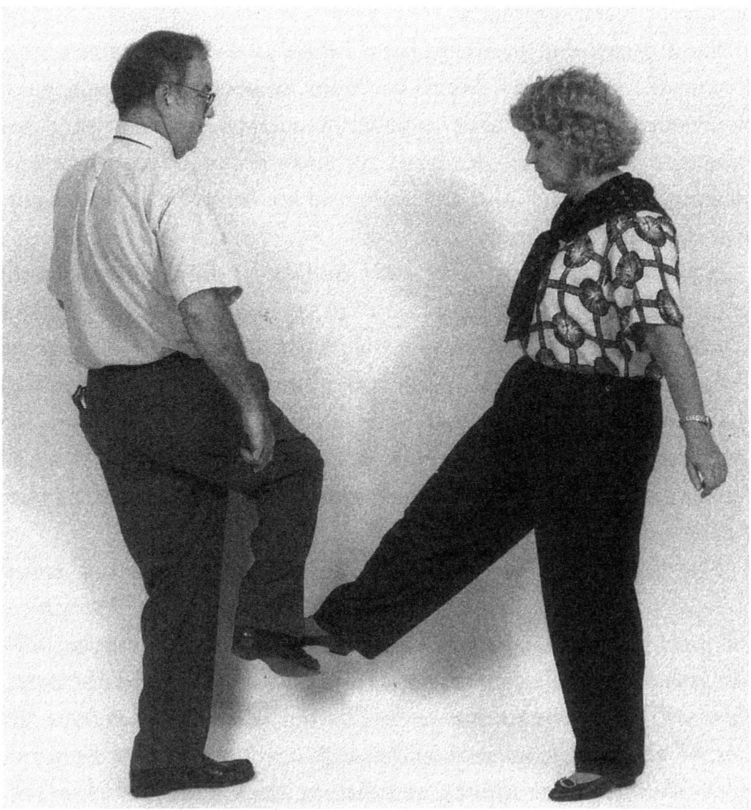

Figure 7-7

TEAM SKILLS

The next major area in the management of the disruptive patient involves the safety of other patients, staff members, and bystanders (Haven & Piscitello, 1989). The escalation of violent behavior is minimized when the staff members clearly know what is expected of them and have had experience and training in dealing with the violent patient, which gives them confidence. Positive and successful interventions demand a coordinated plan of action. Release and control theories are utilized in those incidents that require a team approach.

Some treatment facilities use a "show of force" in an attempt to control "acting out" behavior. Many times a patient will yield to the show of force. But in those situations in which physical intervention becomes necessary, a "show of force" may lack any cohesive leadership and the potential for injury to the patient and the staff is greater.

A team consists of three staff members trained in personal safety skills. Once notified about an emergency, they will meet briefly to familiarize themselves with the situation and to create a plan of action. Preestablished code phrases as a signal for actual "hands on" involvement will be used; for instance, "Will you sit in the green chair?" The team will use every effort to provide the patient with options and face-saving choices to prevent further escalation.

The team will form a triangle around the patient and avoid face-to-face confrontation to minimize intimidation. The stance and personal space concepts discussed earlier in this chapter will be used. Remove other patients and bystanders from the area. This will allow the patient to be further isolated and reduce the "show" element. The team leader will employ verbal techniques in an attempt to set appropriate limits, deescalate the situation, and avoid the use of physical intervention.

The team will physically "flow" with the patient. As the patient moves, the team will move, while maintaining the triad. If the patient begins or continues to escalate in response to the team leader's verbal interaction, another team member will take over, refocus the patient's attention, and provide redirection. Only one member of the team will speak at any one time. "The confidence and control of a well-trained team most likely will be perceived by the patient who is losing control and will provide him or her with a sense of safety" (Haven & Piscitello, 1989). If the patient makes physical contact with a team member, the entire team must react and respond as a unit. This includes premature or accidental contact. A team member should never attempt to handle a situation alone as this can increase the potential for injury to everybody.

Once physical contact has been initiated and the situation unfolds, each team member has a role. A technique called the "lean" will be utilized by two of the team members when the code phrase is said or after physical contact with the patient has occurred.

The "lean" consists of two team members immobilizing one arm each by wrapping both of their arms around the upper part of the patient's arms and leaning onto him or her while shifting as much of their weight as possible. The feet of each of the two team members will be spread approximately a shoulder width apart and will be placed at a 90-degree angle to the midline of the patient. The feet should be planted away from the patient with the legs straight. Do *not* pull on the patient, as the intent is to expend the patient's energy. The third team member will act as a "steering committee." This person will hold the patient's belt or waistband with one hand while placing the other hand on the back, between the patient's shoulders. This individual can either pull or push the patient, which will act as a stabilizing force for the team while adding drag and weight to exhaust the patient. In using a team approach and the lean, no one is actually struggling with the patient, but is providing "dead weight." A patient's ability to support this additional weight is time limited. Once the patient tires and drops to one knee, he or she can be maneuvered into a control position. One team member will stand on each side of the patient with the inside of his or her legs in the patient's armpits. These two team members will hold the patient's wrists with their outer hands while placing their inner hands on the patient's shoulders with downward pressure. The patient's arms are used as levers, with the team members' bodies used as a fulcrum. The steering committee, or third team member, continues to hold the belt or waistband. Verbal techniques continue to be utilized.

If a full takedown becomes necessary, it will be completed in two phases from the control position. In phase 1, the two team members in the control position on the patient's arms will go from the standing position as described above to a one-knee kneeling position (Figure 7-8). On a count of three or at another pre-established sign, the two team members on the arms will roll their outer legs (keeping the toes of those feet on the floor) directly forward and down until the knees are on the floor. The inner legs will remain in the armpit while the patient's arms remain in the leverage position. For completion of phase 2, on an agreed command, rotate the inner leg in a straight, forward roll to the knee (again keeping the toes of that foot on the floor). The steering committee will pull up and back at the belt. At this point, the patient will be flat on his or her stomach. It is recommended not to place a hand under the chin of the patient (as was done in the past), because of the danger of being bitten and the prevalence of the human immunodeficiency virus (HIV). The patient will generally lift his or her head as a reflex when going down. The actions of the steering committee provide some additional protection for the patient.

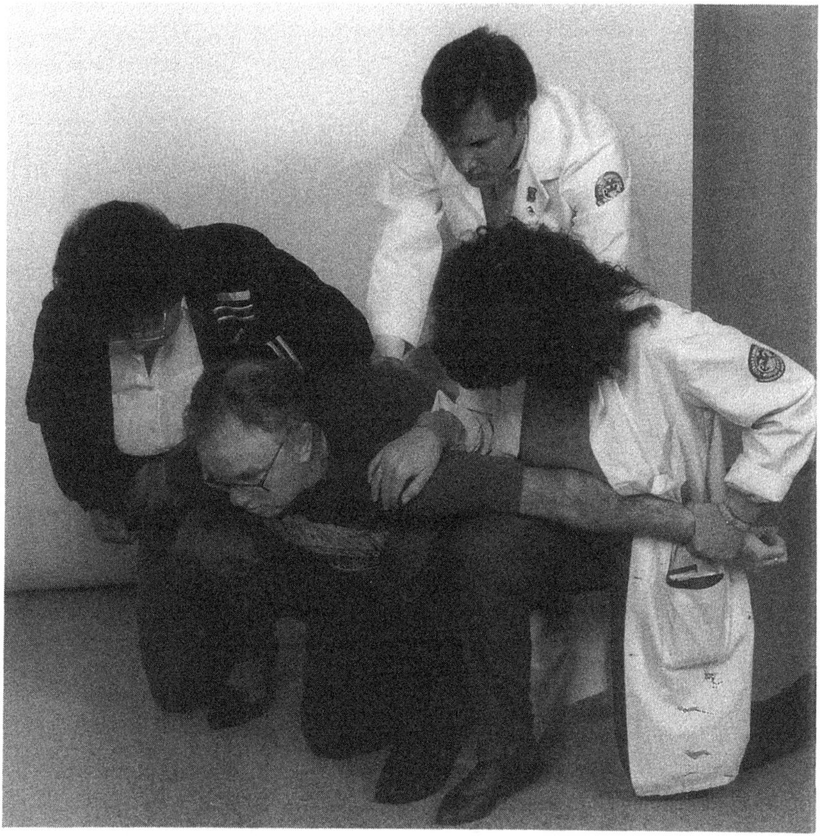

Figure 7-8

After the rolldown, the two team members who maintain the leverage control on the arms will rotate their bodies to assume positions of leaning against the side of the patient and being back to back with each other. In order to control the legs, the third team member will lie over the patient at the level of the buttocks and will roll downward toward the lower legs and feet. That staff member will adjust his or her roll in order to lie across and hold the lower legs and feet of the patient at the end of the maneuver (Figure 7-9). The weight on the patient's legs will prevent the

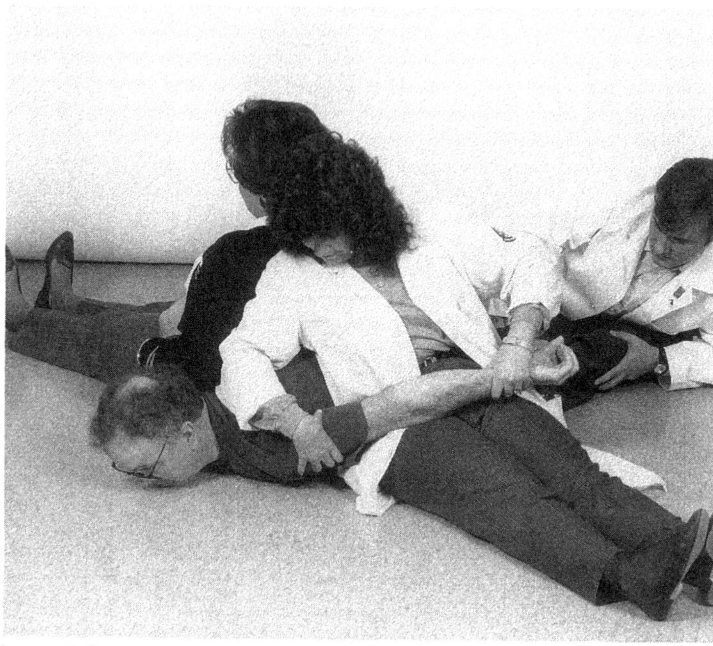

Figure 7-9

use of the patient's feet as an additional weapon. Verbal techniques will continue to be used to defuse the situation.

In this position, the individual can be medicated by injection or placed in leather restraints, prior to removal to another area. Although there are carry positions to transport patients, their use is not encouraged. Once a patient has been placed in leather restraints, he or she can ambulate to another location, if necessary. Four-point restraints will allow some leg movement.

It must be stressed that team techniques require training and experience, as well as a thorough knowledge of personal safety skills. The information outlined indicates the complexity of the team approach. The creation of well-trained response teams at any facility is strongly encouraged.

THE ARMED PATIENT

The last area of discussion is the use of weapons by patients. The term "weapons" refers to any object that can be used to cause harm or threat of harm to self, others, or property. That definition encompasses virtually every physical aspect of the environment. It includes paper, pens, pencils, telephones, typewriters, shoes, soda cans, chairs, tables, belts, and light bulbs. Awareness of the environment and use of the key concepts of prevention are the best countermeasures in this area. Personal safety skills (space and stance) and verbal skills are invaluable. Requests and commands (never threats) can be useful as well. The initial assessment will include the type of weapon being used, the presence of observers, the type of demands and/or threats, psychological aspects, and known history. Attack with a weapon may be a spontaneous or a planned act.

Remember:

- Whenever a weapon is involved, the personal space between the staff member and the patient should be increased. Leave the area and contact the police or security personnel immediately, if possible.
- Use verbal interaction very cautiously since the situation may escalate even further.
- Never threaten the attacker.
- If the weapon is a gun or knife, do whatever is requested.
- Larger objects, such as chairs or large ashcans, can be blocked with similar objects.
- In blocking an object with another object, use the same stance as described earlier. The primary difference is that the width between the legs will be wider, with the weight primarily on the back leg. The blocking object will be presented to the front as a block.

- Don't play hero when a weapon is involved.
- Although forward rolls into a patient and other techniques can be used, they are dangerous and can injure both the patient and the staff member.

CONCLUSION

In summary, prevention is always the primary consideration for managing disruptive or violent behavior. Although many techniques and principles have been discussed, ranging from individual to team skills, any physical confrontation can result in injury to the staff member or the patient. Violence can always occur despite the use of precautions. However, violence is always time limited. Self-confidence generated by the realization that one can provide control is often recognized by the patient. The ability to handle situations based on a knowledge of personal safety skills and team skills can result in a milieu in which disruptive behavior can be controlled or prevented.

REFERENCES

Haven, E., & Piscitello, V. (1989). The patient with violent behavior. In S. Lewis, R. Grainger, W. McDowell, R. Gregory, & R. Messner (Eds.), *Manual of psychosocial nursing intervention* (pp. 187–204). Philadelphia: Saunders.

Veterans Administration (1987) Physical management techniques. From *Prevention and management of disruptive behavior.* A course presented by the Veterans Administration Southeastern Regional Medical Education Center, Birmingham, Ala.

8

Restraint and Seclusion

SUSAN LEWIS,
R.N., C.S., PH.D.

Restraint and seclusion are levels on a continuum of care for psychiatric patients. Although psychotropic medications have reduced the need for restraint and seclusion, instances do occur when these measures are necessary. Care givers are responsible for ensuring patient safety. The law, however, states that patients have a legal right to receive the least restrictive means of treatment. It is the clinician's duty to balance this legal right with safety needs, giving consideration to both the individual patient and the overall treatment milieu.

When an aggressive, potentially dangerous person cannot be reasoned with, persuaded, or managed by less restrictive measures, the use of physical restraint may be necessary to protect that individual and others. If not used with caution and consideration, such measures can increase anxiety, agitation, anger, and confusion. It is wise to keep in mind that even though restraint and seclusion are part of a therapeutic regimen, they do jeopardize the patient's rights, dignity, and privacy.

DEFINITIONS

The term "physical restraints" refers to all appliances that inhibit freedom of movement. Sometimes they are called "patient protective devices" or "supportive devices." There is some difference

Table 8-1

Physical restraints
Supportive devices
Mechanical restraints
Seclusion

in the definition of terms and in the apparatuses themselves (Table 8-1).

Supportive devices are nonlocking devices applied to prevent patients from accidental falls or self-injury. These include soft wrist and ankle restraints, waist restraints, vests, side rails, mittens, and wheelchair restraints. In many treatment settings a physician's order is necessary for use of supportive devices.

Mechanical restraints are mechanisms that, by means of locks of durable construction, impose extreme limitation on the patient's freedom of action. Leather wrist and ankle restraints fall into this category. A physician's order is required for the use of mechanical restraints.

The word *seclusion* refers to a treatment modality whereby the patient is confined to a safe, controlled, and secure environment that has a marked decrease in external stimuli. Seclusion areas are sometimes called "time-out" or "quiet" rooms. A physician's order should be written for seclusion.

INDICATIONS FOR THE USE OF RESTRAINT AND SECLUSION

The need to restrain or seclude should be carefully assessed and documented, although this decision often has to be made quickly. Each clinical setting should have established policies and procedures governing the use of these interventions (Table 8-2).

Table 8-2
Indications for Restraint and Seclusion

1.	Violent behavior—harm to self, others, or property
2.	Disruption of the treatment program
3.	Failure of less restrictive means
4.	As part of prescribed behavioral therapy
5.	Regressed, socially adversive behavior
6.	Patient request
7.	Select medical–surgical problems
8.	Need for decrease in external stimuli
9.	Protection from other patients

Criteria for the use of both restraint and seclusion include:

1. Prevention of serious harm to the health and safety of the patient and/or others. A patient can be dangerous to self through deliberate suicidal acts or other forms of self-injury. The patient who is self-abusive or self-mutilating must be protected from his or her impulses until control is regained.

   Intense excitement or behavioral dyscontrol can lead to exhaustion and injury, as in delirium tremens and physical exhaustion or cardiovascular collapse as a result of hyperactivity (Tardiff, 1989).

   Restraint or seclusion may be used in the presence of marked agitation, thought disorder, or severe confusion in an individual whose medical condition prevents or limits the use of neuroleptic drugs (e.g., severe heart disease, pregnancy, severe tardive dyskinesia) (Tardiff, 1989, p.29).
2. Prevention or serious obstruction, hindrance, or interruption of the treatment program or damage to the physical environment.
3. When other less restrictive measures, such as medication

and interpersonal techniques, have been tried and proved unsuccessful.

4. As a designated aspect of ongoing behavior therapy (Parks, 1990).
5. Limitation of such regressed, socially adversive behavior as smearing stool, conspicious masturbation, destruction of property, and persistent intrusiveness.
6. Patient request. Some patients will ask to be put in restraints or seclusion when they sense a loss of control. Requests for this level of intervention must be carefully evaluated. There are circumstances when the request is inappropriate. For example, when a borderline patient volunteers for seclusion, it may foster regressive, pathological needs. Adolescents and antisocial persons may try to provoke staff members, test limits of tolerance, or impress others with their bravado (Tardiff, 1989).

In some settings, these measures are instituted only after the individual has begun to act out. In other clinical areas, a patient may be secluded or restrained in the process of escalation prior to an incident. In the latter instance, staff members must be very familiar with select patients and must rely on *specific* individual behaviors that have predicted violence in the past, such as increased agitation, glazed eyes, or sexual preoccupation (Tardiff, 1989).

Criteria for Restraint Only

Patients with certain medical–surgical conditions may benefit from the temporary use of supportive devices or restraints. In neurological conditions such as delirium or dementia, or when a confused patient is apt to pull out intravenous and central lines, nasogastric tubes, or Foley catheters, restriction of movement may be warranted.

Criteria for Seclusion Only

There are times when seclusion is the most appropriate and least restrictive means of treatment:

1. When a patient has been sedated but does not sleep and continues to get out of bed, climb over side rails, and wander around or away from the unit.
2. When a patient is becoming overstimulated. The use of seclusion can lessen the disruptive effects of external stimuli, decrease sensory overload, and provide "time out."
3. To protect a patient from possible harm by other patients. Seclusion with close observation can offer safety.

CONTRAINDICATIONS TO RESTRAINT AND SECLUSION

Restraint and seclusion should *never* be used as a substitute for patient care or as a convenience for the staff. Patients in restraints are thought of as being "safer" and less troublesome. But when in restraint or seclusion, they are more vulnerable to a host of complications.

These treatment modalities should not be used for punishment. The punitive use of restraint and seclusion may be covert. Careful rationalizations and skillfully worded progress notes can make their use seem appropriate. One's personal biases and prejudices should not be allowed to influence decisions concerning patient care. Clinical staff members need to be alert to their own feelings and beliefs about violent patients so that these are identified and not acted on.

Patients on neuroleptic medications such as phenothiazines that impair thermoregulation should never be secluded or restrained in a room that cannot be cooled on hot days (Table 8-3).

Table 8-3
Contraindications to Restraint and Seclusion

1.	Staff convenience
2.	Punishment, prejudice
3.	Unknown or unstable medical status
4.	Inability to regulate room temperature

Contraindictions to Seclusion

There are times when seclusion is not recommended and may actually complicate a patient's condition or endanger him or her in some way. Seclusion is not appropriate for patients with an unknown or unstable medical status. This includes patients with delirium of unknown origin, drug overdose, or serious and uncontrolled self-abuse or self-mutilation.

Hazards

Patients placed in restraints are subject to a number of hazards (Table 8-4). They are totally dependent on the care givers to provide even their most basic needs. Being restrained can limit

Table 8-4
Hazards of Restraint and Seclusion

1.	Limited rights
2.	Reduced privacy and dignity
3.	Inhibited mobility, confinement
4.	Restricted breathing
5.	Disorientation
6.	Memory impairment
7.	Impaired circulation and skin integrity
8.	Incontinence
9.	Emotional distress
10.	Vulnerability

rights, reduce privacy, decrease dignity, inhibit mobility, restrict breathing, promote disorientation, impair memory, impair circulation, promote incontinence, cause emotional distress, and increase vulnerability.

PROCEDURES

Staff members should be "tuned in" to the unit dynamics on several levels. Knowledge of patient diagnosis and past history of disruptive behavior can alert the clinician to potential problems. Awareness of patient interactions can give clues to areas of friction. The presence of staff conflict can interfere with patient care and foster disruption.

The use of mechanical restraint constitutes a psychiatric emergency. Every effort should be made to limit the time spent in restraints. Verbal intervention and medication promote the regaining of control. At least 50% of patients will take an oral concentrate (Dubin, Benfield, & Berger, 1981). Parenteral administration of medication can also be used. With intensive intervention, most of these patients can be released from restraint in 90–120 minutes (Dubin et al., 1981).

Patients should be told they are being restrained for their protection and that their safety is a priority. Once a decision to restrain has been made, there should be no negotiation. Enough staff members should be present to carry out the procedure. The clinicians should continue verbal support and inform the patient of each step in the process (Parks, 1990). Use of team contact skills is crucial. The crisis intervention team consists of a minimum of three people with a designated leader and a prearranged plan. Backup should be available. Some authorities prefer a minimum of four or five people, one for each limb and a team leader to direct their efforts. Team skills are discussed in depth elsewhere in this book (Chapter 7).

The procedure calls for restraint of all four limbs and sometimes a belt or vest. Generally, patients are placed on their backs. If delirious because of intoxication or a head injury and likely to vomit, it is possible to restrain a patient in a prone position with the head to one side. These patients require very close monitoring. Restraints themselves should be applied with care. When a patient is placed in restraints, this is the equivalent of an intensive-care situation. The patient at this point requires one-to-one (1:1) observation. It is crucial that staff members assigned to do 1:1 be relieved of other unit duties. It is *not* recommended that a staff member watch two patients at once—1:1 means 1:1. The staff-to-patient ratio should be sufficient to allow this. Attention must also be given to which staff member is assigned to give direct care to the restrained patient. Caring for a patient in restraints is a full-time job. Airway, circulation, skin condition, and mental status must be monitored. Such basic needs as nutrition, elimination, and safety must be considered.

A physician's order is required.

When patients regain control, restraints are released gradually. For example, an arm may be released. Some 15–30 minutes later, the contralateral leg is released, and so on until the patient is allowed up.

SUMMARY

Restraint and seclusion are sometimes necessary to manage violent, assaultive behavior. They should be used with care and consideration for the patient because they do restrict mobility and limit patient rights.

When used with concern and respect for the patient, they can be an effective means of managing disruptive behavior until less restrictive measures such as medication take effect.

REFERENCES

Dubin, W., Benfield, T., & Berger, M. (1981). Management of violent patients. *In Management of violent patients in the community*, a symposium (pp. 3–10). New York: Roerig, a division of Pfizer Pharmaceuticals.

Parks, J. (1990). Violence. In J.R. Hillard (Ed.), *Manual of clinical emergency psychiatry* (pp. 147–160). Washington, D.C.: American Psychiatric Press.

Tardiff, K. (1989). *Concise guide to assessment and management of violent patients*. Washington, D.C.: American Psychiatric Press.

9

Hostage Situations and the Mental Health Professional

THEODORE B. FELDMANN, M.D.
PHILLIP W. JOHNSON, PH.D.

Hostage taking has increased alarmingly in our society. One need only pick up the newspaper to learn of hostage incidents, often with tragic outcomes. For example, during a store robbery in California, 30 people were taken hostage and several eventually were killed during a shoot-out by the hostage takers with police officers. An Indiana high school student who had been suspended for disciplinary reasons returned later on the day of his suspension with several guns and held a classroom of students hostage. A man involved in a worker's compensation case in Alabama became disgruntled with the legal procedures and took a sheriff's deputy hostage in the courthouse to protest the situation. A psychiatric resident at a Veterans Administration Medical Center in Ohio was held hostage for five hours by a patient demanding narcotic medication. Hostage taking has also been used for political leverage on an international level.

These and many other examples illustrate the magnitude of the hostage-taking problem. This chapter examines that problem, describes the motivations for taking hostages, outlines hostage negotiation strategies, and presents guidelines for mental health professionals who are confronted with a hostage incident.

DEFINING THE HOSTAGE SITUATION

The phenomenon of hostage taking has reached epidemic proportions over the past 25 years. A hostage situation may be defined as one in which a person or persons are held against their will, with their release contingent on certain demands being met. Essential to the hostage situation is the presence of demands; without demands a hostage situation does not exist. This is in contrast to a barricade or potential suicide situation in which an individual holds himself or herself, and perhaps others, but makes no demands. In this instance there is no leverage or bargaining point around which release of those held can be obtained.

WHO TAKES HOSTAGES?

The motivations for hostage taking are many but can be summarized as follows: (1) to effect an escape from an interrupted criminal act; (2) to elicit sympathy for radical causes; and (3) to embarrass governments into forcing a change in domestic or foreign policy (Fuselier, 1981; FBI Special Operations and Research Unit, 1981; Stratton, 1978).

A review of case studies by law enforcement officers reveals four categories of persons who take hostages (Fuselier, 1981; Gray, 1981). These include (1) persons with mental disorders, (2) criminals without mental disorders who planned to take hostages in the commission of a crime, or who took hostages because they were interrupted during the crime; (3) prisoners in penal institutions who take hostages in order to escape or to effect some change in the penal system; and (4) terrorists who take hostages in order to secure retribution or the alleviation of disturbing social conditions.

It has generally been considered that the mentally ill group comprises over 50% of all hostage takers (Fuselier, 1981). These persons are thought to represent four traditional diagnostic groups: (1) schizophrenia, (2) depression, (3) antisocial personality disorder, and (4) inadequate personality disorder. This last group corresponds to a DSM-II disorder that is characterized by low self-esteem and inept responses to stress (Strentz, 1983). The inadequate personality may be viewed as related to several of the DSM-III-R personality disorders that are marked by a high degree of impulsivity.

HOSTAGE NEGOTIATIONS: BASIC CONCEPTS

In response to the phenomenon of hostage taking, strategies for hostage negotiation were developed. The main impetus for developing negotiation protocols was the terrorist action against Israeli athletes during the 1972 Munich Olympics (Fuselier, 1981). As a result, law enforcement agencies around the world have been forced to address the hostage taking problem (Vandiver, 1981). When hostage situations occur, law enforcement personnel must establish meaningful contact with hostile, desperate, or mentally ill individuals. In weighing the demands of the hostage takers versus the welfare of the hostages, there is a delicate balance between decisions that involve active and empathic listening and those that eventuate in tactical options (Fuselier, 1986). Because of the high potential for a tragic outcome, a thorough understanding of the dynamics of hostage situations and negotiations is essential.

The basic goals of hostage negotiation may be summarized as follows: (1) to establish contact with the hostage takers; (2) to elicit specific information about the event, including the number of hostages and hostage takers, demands, illness or injury to the hostages, and motivations for the incident; and (3) to conduct a meaningful dialogue with the hostage takers that will result in the surrender of the subjects and the safe release of the hostages. This dialogue may involve a mutual give-and-take in which some demands are met in exchange for the safe release of the hostages (e.g., trading food for the release of hostages). Other demands, such as for weapons or a getaway car, are not met under any circumstances. The overall objective of the negotiations is to obtain the release of the hostages without any injuries to them, law enforcement officers, or hostage takers, and without the use of tactical personnel (e.g., SWAT). These strategies have been described by Fuselier (1981) and others.

THE DYNAMICS OF HOSTAGE SITUATIONS AND NEGOTIATIONS

When the principles of hostage negotiation are compared with those of psychotherapy, certain similarities may be seen. Negotiations, for example, have dynamics similar to therapy. A variety of factors, both internal and external to the hostage situation, influence the progress of the negotiations, just as similar factors influence the course of psychotherapy.

A process that has distinct stages similar to those of psychotherapy may also be observed to develop. These stages include (1) exploration of the problem, for example, how many hostages are being held and what the demands of the hostage taker are; (2) development of a working alliance between the negotiator and hostage taker, essentially an agreement to work together to resolve the situation; (3) working through of goals, in this case, the successful release of the hostages; and (4) termination, which would include the surrender ritual and the release of the hostages. In spite of these similarities, however, it must be remembered that hostage negotiation is not a form of psychotherapy. While many similarities exist, the basic goals of the negotiation are very different from the goals of therapy. It is for this reason that mental health professionals should not serve as negotiators. This is a role best reserved for trained law enforcement officers.

As mentioned previously, the interaction of the negotiator with the hostage taker is a complex phenomenon, not unlike the interaction of a patient with a psychotherapist. Empathy and transference reactions, for example, may be seen as prominent within the negotiations process. In certain hostage situations, the negotiator may become a significant object for the hostage taker. An appreciation of this may be very helpful in guiding the negotiator.

Transference reactions between the hostage taker and the negotiator may also emerge. During negotiations, for example, the hostage taker may experience a desire to become one with the negotiator, thus acquiring strength and stability from the negotiator. The hostage taker may manifest a need for accepting and confirming responses from the negotiator. In other instances, there is an idealization of the negotiator as an all-powerful, benevolent figure. When this occurs, the hostage taker develops an intense trust in the negotiator, wishing to please the negotiator and gain his or her acceptance. At other times, the hostage taker comes to view the negotiator as someone very much like himself or herself, essentially an alter ego. These transferences closely parallel the transferences described in much of the literature on psychotherapy (Wolf, 1988).

The stress of the hostage situation likewise may lead to fragmentation in the hostage taker, the extent of which will be determined in part by the degree of his or her psychopathology. The nature of the hostage situation will also influence the degree of fragmentation. If psychopathology is already present (e.g., the borderline/inadequate hostage taker), this will be more pronounced; however, it should be remembered that extreme stress can lead to fragmentation in any personality (e.g., post-traumatic stress disorder). In response to the fragmentation, certain behaviors may be utilized to restore partial cohesion. This may increase the risk of harm to the hostages, particularly if substance abuse or violence is the primary manifestation.

Empathic responses by the negotiator can decrease the fragmentation and stabilize both the fragmenting personality and the negotiation process. In essence, the negotiator must be able to establish a meaningful relationship with the hostage taker, and utilize that relationship to bring about a successful resolution. In addition, during the course of the negotiation process, the negotiator must also use the relationship to stabilize a potentially explosive situation and to convince the hostage taker that it is in his or her best interest to surrender. Many variables complicate this process, including the criminal or violent tendencies of the hostage taker, the nature of the events that led to the hostage taking in the first place, the degree of ego integrity possessed by the hostage taker, and the skill of the negotiator. Other external variables over which the negotiator may have little control, such as media intrusions or unpredictable behavior by the hostages, will also influence the outcome. Thus the negotiation process is an exceedingly complex one.

MANAGEMENT OF THE HOSTAGE SITUATION

An appreciation of the basic concepts and dynamics of hostage negotiations is important for mental health professionals because there is a high likelihood that they will be involved in such a situation at some point in their professional careers. The very nature of psychiatric patients—their impulsiveness, a tendency to act out, poor coping skills, and an inability to modulate dysphoric feelings—makes them prone to the taking of hostages. The disgruntled patient, for example, who has some grievance with the hospital or therapist may take hostages as a way of expressing those feelings. Psychotherapists or staff members on inpatient units are most likely to be trapped in a hostage situation. Knowing how to behave and to interact with the hostage taker, as well as fully appreciating the efforts and strategies of law enforcement officers to secure one's release, will contribute to the successful resolution of the situation. Mental health professionals also are often called upon by law enforcement to provide consultation to hostage negotiation teams. This is especially true in the case of the mentally ill hostage taker, where law enforcement personnel require expert mental health input in order to plan and conduct the negotiations effectively. It is obviously much better to be prepared should a hostage situation develop than to be caught off guard and unprepared.

When hostage situations arise, it is imperative that the institution have a response plan in place to deal with the incident. Most institutions have disaster-response plans that could be applied to hostage situations. The most important first step when an incident occurs is to call for law enforcement assistance. The FBI strongly supports the notion that only law enforcement officers trained in hostage negotiation techniques should conduct the actual negotiations. Mental health professionals must keep in mind that a hostage situation is a potentially life-threatening situation, and that only law enforcement agencies are equipped to deal with the negotiations and possible tactical options needed to resolve it.

It is never a good idea to negotiate for the release of one's own people. This was exemplified in the 1987 Atlanta prison riot, in which Cuban inmates seized 88 prison employees to protest the inmates' possible deportation to Cuba. This became the largest and most protracted hostage situation in U.S. history. All of the hostages were employed by the U.S. Bureau of Prisons (BOP). It would have been impossible for BOP personnel to conduct negotiations because they knew all of the hostages. The emotional toll on the hostage negotiators would have been too great (Bell, Lanceley, Feldmann, Worley, Fuselier, & Van Zandt, 1991).

Negotiators need to be highly objective if they are to be successful. In this instance, negotiations were conducted by the FBI, resulting in the safe release of all the hostages.

In addition to not being adequately trained to make the difficult decisions that law enforcement officers often confront during hostage situations, there are a number of other pitfalls that mental health professionals must be aware of when dealing with such incidents. One may be described as the "rescue or Lone Ranger syndrome," in which the mental health professional feels uniquely qualified to resolve the situation by virtue of his or her training in psychology and human behavior. While mental health consultation is often important, the successful resolution of a hostage situation requires a high degree of communication and coordination among negotiators, tactical personnel, and command personnel. Again, this is a role best suited for trained law enforcement officers.

It is often tempting to employ psychotherapeutic techniques when dealing with a hostage taker. As indicated earlier, certain similarities do exist between hostage negotiations and psychotherapy. The differences, however, are significant enough to warrant caution in attempting to employ therapeutic techniques. Hostage takers are not patients or clients, even though they may at times display clear evidence of psychopathology. The decisions needed to resolve the situation may run counter to the training and orientation of psychotherapists. While some psychotherapeutic strategies are useful, others simply do not work, or they make the situation worse.

One example of this is the involvement of family members in the negotiation process. While the family may come forward and offer to "resolve" the situation, the high affect levels associated with many family relationships may serve to escalate it. It is important for the police negotiator to have complete control of the negotiation process and to avoid any unexpected external input. This problem is clearly illustrated in the first case example presented at the end of the chapter.

THE ROLE OF ALCOHOL AND DRUGS

Alcohol and drugs are frequently implicated in hostage situations. When they are present, they complicate the situation and significantly increase the risk of a tragic outcome. One reason that alcohol and drugs pose a significant danger during a hostage incident is that they cause a general increase in the level of impulsivity in the hostage takers. This impulsivity may cause the captors to take unnecessary chances that could jeopardize the safety of the hostages. When these substances are added to the already volatile nature of a hostage situation, the potential for injury becomes much greater.

Alcohol also causes impairment in judgment. When under the influence of alcohol or drugs, for example, the hostage taker may have difficulty in realistically evaluating the nature of his or her actions and their consequences. A false sense of confidence or bravado may ensue, which influences the hostage taker to behave in ways he or she might ordinarily resist. This further increases the risk of injury or death to the hostages and law enforcement officers, as well as the hostage taker.

In a related area, the use of alcohol and/or drugs may increase the risk of aggression. The disinhibiting nature of these agents is well known. Rage reactions have been clearly documented for alcohol and for many drugs. When an armed, and potentially dangerous, captor is under the influence of these substances, the threshold for violence is significantly reduced.

Police officers recognize the dangers inherent in responding to domestic arguments or disputes. In most instances, drug or alcohol abuse accompanies a situation where affect levels are already extremely high, greatly exacerbating the volatility of the incident. It is not uncommon, when police arrive at the scene, for one member of the dispute, who is usually armed, to hold the other parties captive as a way of bargaining with the police officers. Of all hostage situations, these are usually the most explosive and have the highest potential for a tragic outcome.

In our study of aircraft hijackers, we found that the chances of injury or death to someone involved were the highest in those incidents that were accompanied by substance abuse (Bell, Lanceley, Feldmann, Johnson, Cheek, & Lewis, 1989). This finding clearly illustrates how the overall index of risk is increased by drug or alcohol use.

Finally, it is extremely difficult to negotiate with an individual who is intoxicated. Clinicians have long recognized that interviews with intoxicated persons yield only limited information; about the only thing that can be assessed is the level of intoxication. That same patient may appear quite different when sober. The same phenomenon occurs in hostage negotiations. Alcohol or drug intoxication adds a significant degree of difficulty to the negotiation process. Case illustration 1 provides a vivid example of this.

THE SUICIDAL HOSTAGE TAKER

In many hostage incidents, depression and suicidal ideation complicate the situation. The taking of hostages may result from feelings of hopelessness or desperation associated with depression. The suicidal hostage taker may hope to be eventually killed by the police, and may even attempt to provoke police officers into shooting. It is essential for the mental health consultant to be aware of this possibility and to look for indicators of depression and suicide. Negotiators must also be comfortable with discussing this material and utilizing crisis intervention techniques to defuse the situation. Both case illustrations at the end of the chapter deal with suicidal hostage takers.

WHEN THE HOSTAGE TAKER IS KNOWN TO THE CLINICIAN

When the hostage taker is known to a mental health professional, such as a current or former patient, a number of considerations, both positive and negative, emerge. One positive point is that the better one knows the individual, the more information can be supplied to the negotiator. If a therapeutic relationship is in place, this can be used to persuade the subject to surrender.

The professional may be placed in the difficult position, however, of disclosing sensitive information, betraying trust, or providing information that may lead to the injury or death of the hostage taker should tactical measures have to be taken. This, in turn, raises the question of confidentiality. In general, when others are placed at significant risk, confidentiality essentially ends (Smith & Meyer, 1987). Law enforcement officers have the legal right to obtain confidential patient records in such instances, and therapists probably have a moral and ethical obligation to assist them in bringing the incident to a peaceful resolution.

Another issue involves the making and breaking of promises to the hostage taker. One must always consider that one may have to deal with the hostage taker again in some other context. Therefore, as a general rule, it is not advisable to make excessive promises that can never be carried out. Once trust is destroyed during this type of incident, it is very hard to restore.

THE STOCKHOLM SYNDROME

The Stockholm syndrome may be defined as an emotional response on the part of persons held hostage in which they develop strong positive feelings toward the captors and simultaneous negative feelings toward the police (Strentz, 1980). This syndrome was first identified in 1973 following a bank robbery in Stockholm, Sweden, in which four female bank employees were held hostage for 131 hours by a pair of armed robbers. Over the course of this incident, the hostages came to believe that their captors were actually protecting them from the police. Two of the hostages went on to develop romantic attachments to the robbers, with one of them eventually marrying one of the subjects.

This phenomenon can be understood as an unconscious reaction to stress in which the victim identifies with the captor as a way of dealing with the stress. It may be considered to be a function of the defense mechanisms of identification with the aggressor and regression. One factor that appears to influence the development of the Stockholm syndrome is time; the longer the hostages are held, the more likely it is that this phenomenon will be observed. The behavior of the hostage takers will also influence its development. Hostage takers who are viewed as relatively benign, or even considerate, are more likely to be identified with in a positive manner. The Stockholm syndrome has been observed in a number of hostage incidents, and may interfere with negotiations since the hostages view police rather than the hostage takers as the real threat.

WHAT TO DO IF TAKEN HOSTAGE

As mentioned earlier, mental health professionals may be at risk for becoming hostages by virtue of the patient populations with which they work. Although the actual incidence of violence among psychiatric patients is low, their impulsiveness, impaired judgment, poor tolerance of frustration, and inability to deal appropriately with dysphoric feelings may lead to the taking of hostages. Thus, it is imperative that mental health professionals become acquainted with the basic guidelines for one's behavior as a hostage.

Perhaps the fundamental guideline for hostages is to remain calm. Although this admittedly is difficult in a highly stressful situation, the hostage should make a conscious attempt to remember this important point. A highly emotional display on the part of the hostage may only serve to create increased anxiety in the hostage taker, often leading to an escalation of impulsive, irrational, or aggressive behavior. A relatively calm stance, on the other hand, may defuse some of the tension and allow the hostage taker to focus on the negotiations to obtain the hostage's release.

A related point is not to do anything that would threaten or provoke the hostage taker. Arguing with the hostage taker, for example, may only increase the person's negative feelings, thus increasing the chances of aggressive action. As long as the hostage taker feels relatively safe, the chances that the hostage will be harmed decrease. Hostage negotiation specialists at the FBI academy in Quantico, Va., argue that hostages should attempt to "blend into their surroundings" and attract as little attention to themselves as possible. This is particularly important in situations in which the hostage takers appear extremely irritable and agitated. Studies of aircraft hijackings reveal that hostages were injured most often when they tried to provoke or overpower the hijackers (Bell et al., 1989).

If one is held hostage, it is advisable to attempt to do whatever the hostage taker says to do. Refusal or attempts to resist will increase the risk for harm. Resistance will also introduce doubt into the hostage taker's mind as to whether the hostage can be trusted. Any hostage taker will be more likely to harm a hostage viewed as threatening or uncooperative than someone who complies with the hostage taker's wishes.

Another useful tactic is to try to personalize the situation as much as possible. For example, one should tell the hostage taker one's name and ask the hostage taker's name. One should share one's feelings with the subject, particularly if they are feelings of fear or anxiety. The effect is to create a personal relationship between the hostage and the hostage taker. A subject who views the hostage as a unique individual, as opposed to a nameless, faceless object, will be much less inclined to do anything that will cause harm or injury.

These basic guidelines will increase the chances of being released unharmed by any captor. The principles outlined here have been utilized by law enforcement officers, airline personnel, and others who are at high risk for being taken hostage.

CASE ILLUSTRATIONS

Case 1

A 34-year-old white male, Mr. E., abducted an 11-year-old boy and proceeded to a motel approximately 120 miles from the boy's home. A motel guest recognized the boy from pictures shown on television and called the local police, who in turn notified the state police and the FBI. Negotiators established a telephone link with the hostage taker's room. The subject stated that he intended to shoot himself in the chest. Negotiations continued throughout the day.

The hostage taker had been charged in the past with sexual molestation and with breaking and entering, and had served time in prison on these charges. He was separated from his wife and had four children, all of whom had recently been placed in foster homes. Prior to the incident, he had been rejected by his ex-wife in an attempt at reconciliation. Records of a psychological evaluation performed on the hostage taker while he was incarcerated were obtained. He was described as of average intelligence but suffering from personality pathology. This was described as paranoid, passive-aggressive, and impulsive. His tolerance of frustration was low and he had difficulty relating to authority figures. He was also described as having a high degree of anger and resentment. There was a preoccupation with sexual issues; these were related primarily to his being sexually abused as a child and also having been sexually molested while in prison. Based on information obtained from these records, a presumptive diagnosis of borderline personality disorder with antisocial traits can be inferred. He had apparently never been psychotic and denied drug use, but he did have a history of alcohol abuse.

The negotiations were unique in that there were no demands on the part of the subject. A number of requests were made and certain deadlines were given, but none of the requests constituted a true demand. When asked to release the hostage, the subject consistently responded that the hostage did not want to leave. No threats against the hostage were ever made. The subject made numerous references to the hostage as being very important to him. In some ways, it seemed that the hostage made him feel good and that he gained a sense of acceptance from the hostage. For this reason, it was clear that it would be very difficult to convince the subject to release his hostage. The subject seemed dependent on the boy for positive empathic responses. Attempts were made to exploit this in the negotiations by replacing the need for the hostage with a need for the negotiator's acceptance. However, the subject refused to respond to the negotiators in the same manner.

The hostage spoke with negotiators on several occasions. He seemed unharmed and fairly calm, although there was considerable fear in his voice. He indicated that he did not wish to come out, indicating that perhaps the subject had told him that the police would harm them if either came out. This suspicion was confirmed later in the evening after the boy was released.

It was clear that the subject was drinking heavily throughout the negotiations. This was demonstrated by his slurred speech, periods of incoherence, and episodes of irritability. Following these periods, he would appear to become very lethargic and somnolent. It was revealed through the negotiations that the subject had large quantities of alcohol and food in the room, making it apparent that he was prepared for an extended siege. It was the consensus of all involved that they should wait out the subject as long as possible, and no tactical intervention was planned.

At one point in the afternoon, the subject began asking to be allowed to talk to his mother. This request was denied, but he continued to verbalize that wish. Reports from the family suggested that it might be the subject's intent to kill himself in front of the mother. Authorities were also fearful that the subject might kill the mother as well, as his relationship with her reportedly was highly conflicted. A tape made by the mother was played, to which the subject responded by becoming angrier and more upset. This confirmed suspicions that the relationship with the mother was highly conflicted.

The negotiators were never able to establish any rapport with the subject, and his mood fluctuated throughout the day. At one point, however, the negotiator took a more confrontational stance. This resulted in the subject's becoming very angry and agitated.

It was clear that the subject was extremely suicidal and was unwilling to surrender under any circumstances. In the late afternoon, he asked to talk to the media, indicating that he wanted to make a statement; he refused to indicate what he wanted to say and access to media was denied.

In the early evening, he appeared to be drinking more heavily. Speech again became slurred and he was unresponsive for extended periods. A period of silence followed, after which a single gunshot was heard. Several seconds later, the boy ran out of the room and was rescued by tactical personnel. When SWAT officers entered the room, they discovered that the subject had shot himself in the chest. Emergency medical personnel arrived on the scene immediately and began administering to the subject, who died a short time later.

Case 2

Mr. D., a 17-year-old white high school senior, entered his high school at approximately 9:00 A.M. armed with a .44 magnum, a .357 magnum, and a 12-gauge shotgun. He fired one shot into the ceiling and ordered the teacher to send the first two rows of students out of the classroom. He then held 11 other students hostage for all or part of the day.

The subject had apparently planned the hostage taking for some time. The incident actually began on the day before when he met a friend to study, but at some point that evening apparently took his friend hostage. The two stayed out all night, going to school the following morning. The group of students held was a mixture of friends and several students whom the hostage taker did not like. He did not make any threats against the hostages, and as the incident progressed, hostages were released in exchange for food, a radio, movies, or simply at their own request. He seemed concerned about the hostages, something that was facilitated by the fact that they were all known to him. Students who were released reported a very relaxed atmosphere in the classroom and said that they talked with the hostage taker the entire time. In fact, many of the students began giving advice to him on how to conduct himself and what kind of demands to make. He frequently put down his guns, and on several occasions unloaded them so that other students could look at them. The released hostages indicated that they did not try to overpower the hostage taker because they liked him and never felt in any danger. Clear evidence of the Stockholm syndrome emerged from this incident.

The only stated demand was to speak to his father, who lived in Florida. He said that he wanted to understand why his father had left him and also why his father had not contributed child support payments for him. By midafternoon, only two hostages remained. They were released at approximately 6:20 P.M. By this point, it was apparent that the hostage taker intended to kill himself. This was confirmed by several notes and book passages found in the subject's room at home by one of the mental health consultants.

The hostage taker lived in a trailer with his maternal grandparents, who were both in their 80s. They were described as overly strict and did not allow the subject to drive or to go out with girls. They had raised him since his parents' divorce when he was three. Both parents now lived in Florida. He visited his mother every summer but had had no contact with his father since the divorce.

The previous summer he had visited Florida to see his mother and apparently worked there. The money he earned from that job was used to buy his weapons.

He was an honor student and had an IQ tested at 130. He also played in the high school band. Over the past year, his grades had declined, and he became more withdrawn and began to neglect his appearance. Although he had several close friends, most students described him as shy, quiet, and a loner. His grandparents did not allow him to date, but other friends reported that he also had no interest in girls. Classmates said that he became more involved with fantasy material, usually that with a violent theme. He had started reading violence-oriented books and also became more preoccupied with music, particularly heavy metal. While these bands are popular with many teenagers, the hostage taker seemed to take an excessive interest in the lyrics of songs that had violent, sadomasochistic, or suicidal overtones. He would often focus on segments of lyrics taken out of context and attach special meanings to them. His primary interest centered on firearms, and he often went hunting with his friends. This appeared to be his main social activity. Friends talked about his being very knowledgeable about guns and being an excellent marksman.

In spite of the rather relaxed initial atmosphere in the classroom, the hostage taker refused to emerge, and also refused to discuss why he wanted to see his father. As more information was obtained from family and friends, it was felt that the subject might attempt to kill his father and/or himself. It was also felt that he might attempt to provoke the police into killing him. The grandfather reported that over a number of years the subject had developed an intense hatred of the father and the grandfather felt certain that he would kill him if he had the chance. Several friends also reported that. For at least the past year, he had talked to friends about either taking hostages at school or robbing a bank to obtain enough money to go to Florida to kill his father. No one took these threats seriously, and many friends thought that he was joking. He also apparently made a number of contingency plans for the hostage taking in the event that something were to go wrong.

The clinical picture that begins to appear seems consistent with the prodromal signs of a first schizophrenic break or a psychotic depression. He had no psychiatric history, but had apparently mentioned suicide to his friends. A series of poems found in his room all had suicidal references, as well as a rather mystical, bizarre quality. Subsequent psychiatric evaluation confirmed the diagnosis of major depression with psychotic features.

From the outset, he talked openly to the state police negotiator and a good rapport was established. In spite of that rapport, however, the mental health consultants had trouble getting the negotiator to address the issue of suicide directly. He seemed very reluctant to use the words "kill yourself," or "suicide." After some urging, however, he was able to discuss this directly with the subject. This opened up the young man, who seemed relieved to know that someone understood how he felt. The negotiator was able to contract with the subject not to harm himself, and after several minutes, the subject surrendered. He was referred for psychiatric evaluation. It was interesting to note that when he came out, he looked very different from recent pictures. His appearance had deteriorated and he was dressed primarily in black. Subsequent psychiatric examination confirmed a diagnosis of major depression with psychotic features. The subject was referred for psychiatric hospitalization and no charges were pressed.

REFERENCES

Bell, R.A., Lanceley, F.J., Feldmann, T.B., Johnson, P.W., Cheek, C., & Lewis, C.E. (1989). Improving hostage negotiation strategies: An empirical study of aircraft hijackers. *American Journal of Preventive Psychiatry and Neurology, 2*(1), 1–5.

Bell, R.A., Lanceley, F.J., Feldmann, T.B., Worley, T.H., Fuselier, G.D., & Van Zandt, C. (1991). Hostage negotiations and mental health: Experiences from the Atlanta prison riot. *American Journal of Preventive Psychiatry and Neurology, 3*(2), 8–11.

FBI Special Operations and Research Unit (1981). A terrorist organizational profile: A psychological role model. In Y. Alexander & J. Gleason (Eds.), *Behavioral and quantitative perspectives on terrorism.* New York: Pergamon.

Fuselier, G.D. (1981). A practical overview of hostage negotiations. *FBI Law Enforcement Bulletin, 50*(6), 2–11.

Fuselier, G.D. (1986). What every negotiator would like his chief to know. *FBI Law Enforcement Bulletin, 55*(3), 12–15.

Gray, O.M. (1981). Hostage negotiations. *Texas Police Journal, 29*(11), 14–18.

Smith, S.R., & Meyer, R.G. (1987). *Law, behavior, and mental health.* New York: New York University Press.

Stratton, J.G. (1978). The terrorist act of hostage-taking: Exploring the motivation and cause. *Journal of Police Science and Administration, 6*(1), 1–9.

Strentz, T. (1980). The Stockholm syndrome: Law enforcement policy and ego defenses of the hostage. In F. Wright, C. Bahn, & R.W. Rieber (Eds), *Forensic psychiatry and psychology.* New York: New York Academy of Sciences.

Strentz, T. (1983). The inadequate personality as hostage-taker. *Journal of Police Science and Administration, 11*(3), 363–368.

Vandiver, J.V. (1981). Hostage situations require preparedness. *Law and Order,* Sept., 66–69.

Wolf, E.S. (1988). *Treating the self: Elements of clinical self psychology.* New York: Guilford.

10

Institutional Responses to Violent Incidents

DANIELLE M. TURNS, M.D.

Violent incidents are widely underreported in hospitals. While dangerous episodes that do not result in personal injuries are usually taken casually, attacks involving weapons, injuries, or death generate great turmoil. Shock, concern, anger, and guilt feelings are universal and often are mingled with doubts that the incident could have been avoided. Alternatively, inquiries are made suggesting that the matter was not "handled right." Questioning one's own or others' competence brings uncomfortable fears of vulnerability, damaged self-esteem, and impotent rage.

There are little data on how exposure to violence affects the staff or the institution. Transfers to closed wards, treatment with neuroleptics, discharges, and home leaves are minimally affected, primarily due to a hospital administration's open and supportive management (Turns & Gruenberg, 1973). Employees who are victims of patient attacks can develop a post traumatic stress disorder (PTSD)–like syndrome (Engel & Marsh, 1986). A frequent complaint about working conditions is the risk of physical assault and the pervasive impression that nothing is ever done to provide staff protection.

In psychiatry's early days, the hospital setting was architecturally conceived to enhance safety. Treatment facilities used physical confinement for the prevention of violence, unfortunately to excess. Institutions should now, for safety reasons, continue to pay attention to those physical features that may be utilized by patients to harm themselves or others. Currently, isolated offices, the absence of alarm systems (particularly in outpatient settings), and the lack of escape routes are still frequently encountered.

Because of the rising concern about patient assaults on staff members, hospitals in recent times have taken steps to prevent and to deal with the aftermath of violence. Such measures can be broadly classified in five categories: environmental safety precautions, psychological audits or reviews, training programs for employees, counseling for the victims, and legal actions.

ENVIRONMENT SAFETY MEASURES

Alarm systems are prevalent in hospital wards but much less so in outpatient clinics or private offices. The latter two settings are probably more dangerous because of the relative isolation of the therapist. Doctors are often reluctant to request such devices, not only because of feelings of invulnerability, but also because they do not want to appear overly concerned about their patients' potential for violence. Alarms should be incorporated in the design of *all* facilities. They do not offer full protection though, because people often fail to use them even when they sense danger. Only 20% of offices have security systems in place (Dubin, Wilson, & Mercer, 1988). Educational programs should pay attention to that issue and emphasize a "better safe than sorry" philosophy.

Emergency rooms are very dangerous areas. Of patients entering an emergency room, 8% carry weapons (Anderson, Ghali, & Bansil, 1989). Some have chosen to install magnetic screening devices such as those used in airports to identify weapon carriers. Other facilities have instituted a routine for the admission of psychiatric patients that includes a thorough search and a change into hospital clothes prior to entering the ward. Even though these precautions may not appear to foster rapport with a patient, their safety dividend cannot be overlooked. Systematically flagging violent patients' charts and computer files provides a valuable warning to personnel unacquainted with them.

SYSTEMATIC AUDITS

The systematic review of incidents involving physical violence plays a triple role. First, it attracts the attention of the administrators and makes them aware of the extent of the problem. Second, it provides a tool for the identification of risks. One may discover such risks as the physical structure, nonadherence to admission procedure, and/or failure to recognize impending danger and take appropriate action. Last, they permit the identification of patients with violent behavior and alert the staff to potential crises.

Audits are useful in revealing systemic problem patterns. They also may identify weaknesses in prevention and management that must be remedied. Care is taken not to use the results of such audits in what could be perceived as "fault finding." Monitoring of incidents over time provides a gauge of how successful preventive programs are and an indication of what might be changed to achieve even better results.

TRAINING PROGRAMS FOR EMPLOYEES

In-service education should integrate technical learning and exploration of the employees' feelings when confronted with violence. Most educational programs focus on the recognition of danger signals, prevention and verbal techniques, procedures to follow when the situation escalates, and physical management designed to protect the staff and control the patient without causing harm. Such techniques are described elsewhere in this book.

Teaching programs addressing physical management need to be presented regularly so that an employee's response becomes automatic. In most settings, those skills are not used frequently, and thus they may be quickly forgotten. Such workshops are offered on a yearly or biyearly basis. Frequent practice will heighten the person's skill for a time of crisis. New personnel should be trained during their orientation and all staff members, even those not involved in direct patient care, should be involved.

Receptionists are often the first to be approached by an agitated patient, and even maintenance workers, for example, are not immune to attacks. Programs for all employees are cumbersome if only a few trainers are available. A "train the trainers" program can be advantageous, allowing for more frequent sessions with a smaller number of persons at each class.

COUNSELING PROGRAMS FOR EMPLOYEE VICTIMS OF VIOLENCE

People who are victims of violence often tend to minimize the seriousness of incidents, particularly if there is no physical harm. Even when a staff member is injured, there are no formal procedures by which to ventilate feelings or seek advice. Programs should mandate immediate medical and emotional care, legal and practical advice, and follow-up treatment. Provision of psychosocial counseling and a documented investigation of the incident are also important for morale (Engels & Marsh, 1986). Treatment should focus on acute post-traumatic symptoms, anxiety, phobic responses, and dealing with co-workers' reactions to the incident.

There is a tendency to blame the staff and not to support legal charges in order to avoid institutional publicity. An Assaulted Staff Action Program (ASAP) in a state hospital has been successful (Flannery, Fulton, Tausch, & Deloffi, 1991). The ASAP team consists of voluntary clinicians who respond to all assaults, debrief the victim, and arrange for follow-up care. Ongoing interviews are also offered, and a short-term support group meeting is held weekly for victims of violence. The employee's participation is voluntary and the information confidential. Further research will evaluate the therapeutic efficacy and cost-effectiveness of such offerings.

LEGAL ACTIONS

Any institution needs the assistance and expertise of legal counselors to deal with violence in and outside the hospital setting. This is discussed in Chapter 11 on legal issues.

REFERENCES

Anderson, A.A., Ghali, A.Y., & Bansil, R.K. (1989). Weapon carrying among patients in a psychiatric emergency room. *Hospital and Community Psychiatry, 40*(8), 845–847.

Dubin, W.R., Wilson, S.J., & Mercer, C. (1988). Assaults against psychiatrists in outpatient settings. *Journal of Clinical Psychiatry, 49*(9), 338–345.

Engel, F., & Marsh, S. (1986). Helping the employee victim of violence in hospitals. *Hospital and Community Psychiatry, 37*(2) 159–162.

Flannery, R.B., Fulton, P., Tausch, J., & DeLoffi, A.Y. (1991). A program to help staff cope with psychological sequellae of assaults by patients. *Hospital and Community Psychiatry, 42*(9), 935–938.

Turns, D., & Gruenberg, E. (1973). An attendant is murdered: The state hospital responds. *Psychiatric Quarterly, 47*(4), 487–494.

11

Legal Issues

ANTHONY G. BELAK, J.D.
DAVID BUSSE, J.D.

OVERVIEW

A clinician can be held liable in the care of a violent patient when there is proof of a "duty of care owed," a breach of that duty, and some injury to the patient or a third party as a result.

Liability may be based on any number of criteria, such as negligence, battery, lack of informed consent, abandonment, misdiagnosis, or any violation of the many duties owed to the patient. Noncompetent or violent patients retain all the rights and protections of any other psychiatric patient, and often even more responsibilities are imposed on the psychotherapist in these cases.

Therapeutic issues remain confidential even when the patient is violent, except as to the duty to warn *identified* victims or to take the necessary steps to protect the patient or others from his or her violence. The psychotherapist should violate that trust only when professionally or legally required and permitted.

Harm to Self

The psychotherapist has the duty to protect the patient against foreseeable harm, including suicide or self-inflicted injuries. The determining factor is the *reasonable anticipation* or *foreseeability* of the patient's self-inflicted wound. If the individual has been diagnosed as suicidal, reasonable measures must be taken to prevent harm. It is usually up to the jury to decide whether a psychotherapist knew or should have known that a patient was a suicide risk.

Any measures to protect the suicidal person depend on the dangers posed and the foreseeability of self-inflicted injury. A patient with strong suicidal tendencies requires constant observation in an environment free of implements of self destruction. Courts are not receptive to the defense that the patient's contributory negligence caused the injury, and it is irrelevant whether or not the patient's suicidal gestures were "genuine" or "manipulative" (*Cowan v. Deering*, 1987).

All patients must be treated according to similar standards even if the patients are difficult or violent. The professional must, in good faith, take or attempt the actions required to treat or maintain the violent patient within the proper standards of the profession. Informed consent should be obtained from the patient or a surrogate if needed. Consultations should be requested whenever indicated.

Harm to Others

All psychiatric patients, the violent and/or involuntarily committed included, retain the capacity to make informed judgments about their own care and treatment. The psychotherapist has the responsibility to disclose any proposed treatment, its risks and benefits and/or other alternatives, except for life-threatening emergencies. A person cannot be forced to undergo treatment against his or her will unless there is a judicial declaration of incompetence or a crisis that poses an immediate danger of harm to self or others, even when the treatment is considered to be in the best interest of the patient (*Grundy v. Pauley,* 1981). This is appropriate and right in legal theory.

It is not correct for health-care providers to declare an emergency simply because it would be in their own best interests to contain or restrain a violent person. However, when the safety of the patient or others is in jeopardy but no life-threatening situation exists, health-care personnel can partially and in a limited fashion violate the rights of a violent patient. Nonconsensual treatment should be contemplated only when judicial intervention is not practical and some ethics evaluation has been conducted through interdisciplinary judgments.

A recurring pattern of such treatment is not professionally or legally acceptable. All psychiatric patients have the same rights, but those rights and dignities must always be balanced with societal interests and the rights of others.

When the clinician has subdued a hostile patient without the benefit of a court order or informed consent, it is advisable to initiate involuntary hospitalization proceedings even if the patient becomes compliant. Failure to do so exposes the doctor to possible charges of false imprisonment, battery, or violation of informed consent.

Duty to Protect

A psychiatric institution has a duty to protect patients and visitors from foreseeable injuries. That duty is based on the anticipation of injury.

If the hospital personnel know or may know of the patient's violent propensities and do not take adequate precautions, liability for injuries or property damage may be established. The hospital has a duty to segregate a violent patient from the rest of the population or closely to supervise that patient's activities (*Rathbun v. Starr Commonwealth for Boys*, 1985).

Inpatient Versus Outpatient

The psychotherapist's duty to an outpatient differs from that owed to an institutionalized patient. The duty of the hospital is to exercise reasonable care and to safeguard the patient from any known or foreseeable mental or physical condition. That same degree of control cannot be exercised over an outpatient. The doctor is bound only to exercise the degree of professional ability ordinarily utilized by other psychotherapists under similar circumstances in the same or similar communities (*Speer v. United States*, 1982). The relationship between the custodial patient and the doctor differs from a relationship with an outpatient. The therapist of a custodial patient is better able to anticipate potential harm to a particular victim or class of victims. But, as a matter of law, the mere fact that a patient is seen on an outpatient basis does not render future acts unforeseeable.

Generally, expert testimony is required to establish the standard of care and any violation thereof is psychotherapist malpractice. An exception to the rule has been recognized where the lack of care and/or skills is so apparent as to be within the comprehension of the average lay person and requires only common knowledge and experience to understand (*Rosemont, Ins. v. Marshall*, 1986). As one court said, "The test of whether expert testimony is required is whether the matter to be dealt with is so esoteric that jurors of common knowledge and experience cannot form a valid judgment as to whether the conduct of the parties is reasonable" (*Roettfer v. United Hospitals of St. Paul*, 1986).

A psychotherapist ordinarily must testify to the proper standard of care, but that standard may be established by other medical practitioners who are knowledgeable about psychiatric practices or where the standard at issue is one of general medical practice. Otherwise, a general physician or a specialist in a particular field other that psychiatry is not qualified to testify as to the standard of care applicable to psychiatrists. Nonmedical experts, such as psychologists, are competent to testify regarding matters within their fields of knowledge, but not on issues or standards requiring medical knowledge.

INVOLUNTARY COMMITMENT PROCESS

The various state statutes setting forth the process for involuntary commitment are relevant to the issue of legal implications in treating the violent patient. Typically, such statutes will outline the process for hospitalizing patients who otherwise are unwilling to remain in a treatment setting. In the case of the violent or psychotic patient, there is frequently a very thin line separating voluntary from involuntary. Indeed, some may begin their treatment as voluntary, but, because of a refusal to cooperate with treatment, a stagnancy in their medical condition, or a lack of compliance, may migrate from a voluntary to an involuntary status. It is in these situations that the mental inquest commitment statutes and the protection they afford should be reviewed by any medical-care professional who deals with violent patients.

Mental commitment laws provide standards for the medical evidence necessary to maintain a patient in a hospital setting and time limits in which to review the patient's care. In many instances, they also contain statutes outlining the rights of hospitalized patients and special provisions for court review or de novo hearings when a patient refuses aspects of the individualized treatment program.

The use of mental commitment statutes also insulates the hospital against any charges based on the legal doctrine of informed consent or false imprisonment (*Rogers v. Okin*, 1979). The opposite is true if facts emerge to demonstrate that a judicial or court order commitment should have been pursued and for some reason was not.

There are specific instances in which the protection of a court order can be useful in defending the legal consequences of treatment of a violent patient. Nevertheless, a mental commitment judge may order the patient released for lack of sufficient evidence to hold him or her in treatment.

Courts that review the requirements of mental commitment statutes are aware of the balancing process necessary in any decision to hospitalize involuntarily versus to discharge a patient who is borderline dangerous (*Kendall v. True*, 1975).

The right to refuse treatment is not absolute, it is subject to the police power of the state to control persons who are immediate dangers to others or are incompetent and/or unable to care for themselves. However, courts have held that unless there is a judicial declaration of incompetency or an emergency posing an immediate danger to the self or others, a person cannot be compelled to undergo treatment (*Grundy v. Pauley*, 1981). This is the case even if the medical staff members believe the treatment would have been in the best interest of the patient. The de novo hearings mentioned earlier are used when involuntary patients refuse specific parts of treatment. The same provisions come into play when a voluntary patient refuses treatment under those or similar circumstances. Courts historically have allowed some autonomy to what are typically called treatment or hospital review committees. These are given a specified period in which to review a patient's refusal to participate in an aspect of the treatment plan. If no acceptable resolution is reached, the hospital may petition the court to have the patient be required to comply with the treatment in question. The court may consider several factors:

1. The necessity to protect this or other patients from harm.
2. The patient's ability to give informed consent for treatment.
3. The existence of any less restrictive alternative treatments.
4. The risk of side effects from the treatment as proposed.

The advantage of the de novo hearing in the court process is clear. It serves to insulate a medical center from liability for a specific treatment even in cases where a patient is most resistive. The difficulty with a legal provision of this type is the delay factor prior to commencing treatment for a patient who is in dire need of care. Provisions of this type are not intended to override emergency-care provisions for administering treatment or restraint.

DUTY TO WARN OR PROTECT

In 1976 the landmark case of *Tarasoff v. Regents of the University of California* had a major impact on the mental health profession. This decision, now a part of common law, radically altered the concept of confidentiality. Psychiatric practitioners are required to warn victims when dangerous threats are made by their patients. Hence, clinicians must balance the open and confidential communication necessary for proper therapy against the danger to third parties. "The protective privilege ends where the public peril begins" (*Tarasoff v. Regents of the University of California*, 1976).

Under this ruling, the threats must be specific and the victims readily identifiable. During the course of therapy, the mere fact that a patient expresses an intention or desire to harm someone does not, in and of itself, require the psychotherapist to warn the intended victim or take precautionary steps. This obligation is measured by the particular facts and the prevailing standards. Before an agency, hospital, or practitioner incurs a duty to warn, the patient must present a "serious danger of violence" to a foreseeable victim of that danger" (*White v. United States*, 1986).

RECORD-KEEPING ISSUES

A frequent issue in record keeping is whether there is an "appearance of an impropriety" in the care of a particular patient. Unfortunately, even an appearance may give rise to an inference of liability by a court.

In the treatment of a violent or dangerous patient, the medical record affects legal liability in several areas. A failure to review all available treatment records prior to the discharge of a patient can be the basis for a legal action against a physician or a medical center. Supplementary opinions in the medical record by collateral staff members such as psychologists, social workers, and nurses frequently may mark the difference between a finding of an adequate medical record and of reasonable medical decision-making liability.

On the whole, a well-documented medical record will provide better defense of a legal claim against a physician or medical center, even in those instances where the record displays obvious weaknesses in the care of a patient. This is true because of the frequent delays in the bringing of medical malpractice cases and the delay following the initiation of the lawsuit. During those periods of delay, it well may be that the only timely and preserved recollection that one has of a specific prior event is that contained in the sufficient or insufficient entries of a medical record.

LIABILITY OF THE VIOLENT PATIENT

Psychiatric patients, like others, are responsible for the consequences of their acts within the civil justice system and may not escape liability in the event of injury to innocent third parties. Incompetent patients have rights, but along with those rights come commensurate responsibilities. Nevertheless, injured parties usually prefer to bring an action against the health-care provider owing to financial considerations. The health-care provider has remedies against the violent patient for negligent or criminal acts within the clinical setting. The state will prosecute criminal charges brought against a patient who injures someone in the health-care setting. Defendants who are incompetent at the time of trial will not face charges until a later date, because due process requires their full participation in their defense. Depending on the severity of the crime or injury, the prosecutor may or may not take an aggressive approach and place the patient in prison. The question of whether prison is the proper therapy for the violent patient is debated after a crime has been committed and the state becomes involved.

Once a staff member initiates a criminal charge against a patient, a process that is not easy to undo or reverse, the state becomes the party in interest or the party that controls the litigation. At that time, the clinician must be prepared to stop the treatment. This would be primarily a consideration in misdemeanor charges; felony indictments are much more serious. Many states allow for jury verdicts of insane but guilty, and convicted persons are usually confined in secured psychiatric facilities.

An often effective approach to balance the interests of clinicians with their concern for the activities of violent patients, when no serious or permanent harm has resulted, is restitution and probation. In exchange for a guilty plea, held in abeyance, the patient/defendant must indemnify the injured health-care giver for the costs associated with the attack and injury. The patient/defendant must not incur another arrest during a defined period, must pay the victim actual damages for the injury, and may be obligated to make certain promises or meet certain stipulations, such as not seeking treatment with a specific person or in a specific place. Should the patient/defendant violate any of the provisions of a probated sentence, the recourse is incarceration for the balance of the probation period.

If the health-care provider desires monetary damages for physical or emotional injuries, a civil lawsuit may be filed. The clinician must initiate the litigation, absorbing all costs associated therewith, and be prepared for all possible defenses, chief among which is assumption of the risk. People who work with violent persons must be aware of the potential for injury or bodily harm. A severely injured clinician may retort that his or her expectations were exceeded and that the patient maliciously and intentionally caused the injury. Liability may lie with the violent patient following the presentation of evidence at a trial. The clinician should be present and participate in the preparation for trial.

Serious injury usually results in worker's compensation benefits, which is an expeditious and speedy recourse (civil charges may take years to come to trial). If a clinician prevails over a patient in a civil trial for injuries sustained, the clinician may have to reimburse the employer or worker's compensation insurance carrier for the monies expended on those injuries. Even though there may be a remedy, one must employ prudence and research the costs, emotional and monetary, associated with pursuing the day in court. Often, a violent patient may be judgmentproof, which means that any monetary award suggested at trial has little or no hope of being satisfied. The violent patient may not have assets with which to pay damages. Where there are assets, the clinician is well advised to consider some alternative dispute resolution. Mediation is a process whereby a neutral person facilitates, by agreement of the parties, the resolution of any claims. This process is both speedy and private.

Should the patient become injured by the health-care provider following a violent outburst by the patient, can the caregiver be considered liable? The answer is that health-care providers have a duty to protect and keep safe patients and visitors to a facility where people receive medical or psychiatric care. Incompetent patients are owed a higher duty of protection.

If the caregiver knows or should know of the violent propensities or history of a patient and takes no reasonable step to prevent or reduce the impact of a violent act, liability for injury to the patient may rest with the caregiver. Even though a violent outburst may not have been foreseeable and reasonable precautions were taken, liability may follow if the caregiver uses unreasonable force to subdue a violent patient. The standard is what another caregiver would have done under like or similar circumstances—"the reasonable person test." The result will depend on the testimony of other professionals. Expert opinions are required to find a deviation from the standard of care.

The first test for deviation from the standard of care is whether the policy of the institution was followed. It is considered negligent not to follow the guidelines established by policies, and, if an injury results, liability will often be attributed to the caregiver. A per se violation of the established policy immediately shifts the burden to the care provider to explain why any deviation should not be considered negligence. Such policies are intended physically to protect the patient and staff from injury, but when injury occurs and money damages are requested, what protections are there against legal liability? A basic rule is that policies cannot be written for every perceived situation, and a sound policy is a simple rule that allows for judgmental decision making, instantaneously, under the circumstances. To support a best-judgment policy, proper training for and by decision makers is crucial. So long as a professional health-care provider is apprised of all available facts and information and uses his or her best judgment, negligence may not be found; however, substantial deviation from a formal policy brings an automatic charge of negligence.

STANDARD OF CARE

Providers of psychiatric treatment have a legal obligation to maintain a certain quality or *standard of care*. In order to determine a particular standard of care, three sources are considered. Court decisions are the main source of legal standards in medical cases. The findings of courts as to liability help to establish the standard of care owed to a particular patient under particular circumstances. Another source is the testimony of appropriate clinical experts in a given situation. Finally standard of care is found in laws, regulations, manuals, memoranda, policies, and other written documents pertaining to the issues before the court. There is a hierarchy of value according to which these elements are weighed. Thus federal, state, and local laws are given higher priority than federal or state regulations and local institutional policy.

CONCLUSION

The legal implications involved in treating psychiatric patients are numerous and complex. Not only are clinicians legally responsible for matters relating to the medical care of patients in general, but they also must be concerned about issues specific to psychiatric patients. Violence or the potential for violence poses additional complications. Health-care professionals are being held accountable to an ever-increasing degree for the actions of their patients. Awareness and understanding of legal issues are imperative for all practitioners.

REFERENCES

Cowan v. Deering, 215 N.J. Super. 484, 55 2A. 2d 444 (1987).
Grundy v. Pauley, 619 S.W. 2d. 730 (Ky. App. 1981).
Kendall v. True, 391 F. Supp. 413 (D.C. Ky. 1975). Minimum requirements

of due process for involuntary commitment of a mentally ill person are a right to a preliminary probable-cause hearing, a right to notice before a final hearing, a holding of a final hearing within 21 days of initial confinement, and the right of the patient to be present at both hearings; see page 414.

Rathbun v. Starr Commonwealth for Boys, 145 Mich. App. 303, 377 N.W. 2d. 872 (1985).

Roettfer v. United Hospitals of St. Paul, 380 N.W. 2d. 856 (Minn. App. 1986).

Rogers v. Okin, 478 F. Supp. 1342 (D.C. Mass. 1979).

Rosemont, Ins. v. Marshall, 481 So. 2d. 1126 (Ala. 1986).

Speer v. United States, 512 F. Supp. 670 (N.D. Tex. 1981), Aff'd, 675 F. 2d. 100 (5th Cir. 1982).

Tarasoff v. Regents of the University of California, 17 Cal. 3d. at 436, 131 Cal. Rptr. at 24, 551 P. 2d. at 334 (1976).

White v. United States, 780 F. 2d. 97 (D.C. Cir. 1986).

Name Index

Subject Index

For Product Safety Concerns and Information please contact our EU representative GPSR@taylorandfrancis.com
Taylor & Francis Verlag GmbH, Kaufingerstraße 24, 80331 München, Germany

www.ingramcontent.com/pod-product-compliance
Ingram Content Group UK Ltd.
Pitfield, Milton Keynes, MK11 3LW, UK
UKHW021244190926
475569UK00001BA/3

* 9 7 8 1 1 3 8 1 6 5 9 3 9 *